IMPROVING SURFACE TRANSPORTATION SECURITY

A Research and Development Strategy

Committee on R&D Strategies to Improve Surface Transportation Security

National Materials Advisory Board
Commission on Engineering and Technical Systems

Computer Science and Telecommunications Board
Commission on Physical Sciences, Mathematics, and Applications

Transportation Research Board

National Research Council

NATIONAL ACADEMY PRESS
Washington, D.C.

NATIONAL ACADEMY PRESS • 2101 Constitution Avenue, N.W. • Washington, D.C. 20418

NOTICE: The project that is the subject of this report was approved by the Governing Board of the National Research Council, whose members are drawn from the councils of the National Academy of Sciences, the National Academy of Engineering, and the Institute of Medicine. The members of the panel responsible for the report were chosen for their special competences and with regard for appropriate balance.

The National Academy of Sciences is a private, nonprofit, self-perpetuating society of distinguished scholars engaged in scientific and engineering research, dedicated to the furtherance of science and technology and to their use for the general welfare. Upon the authority of the charter granted to it by Congress in 1863, the Academy has a mandate that requires it to advise the federal government on scientific and technical matters. Dr. Bruce Alberts is president of the National Academy of Sciences.

The National Academy of Engineering was established in 1964, under the charter of the National Academy of Sciences, as a parallel organization of outstanding engineers. It is autonomous in its administration and in the selection of its members, sharing with the National Academy of Sciences the responsibility for advising the federal government. The National Academy of Engineering also sponsors engineering programs aimed at meeting national needs, encourages education and research, and recognizes the superior achievements of engineers. Dr. William A. Wulf is president of the National Academy of Engineering.

The Institute of Medicine was established in 1970 by the National Academy of Sciences to secure the services of eminent members of appropriate professions in the examination of policy matters pertaining to the health of the public. The Institute acts under the responsibility given to the National Academy of Sciences by its congressional charter to be an adviser to the federal government and, upon its own initiative, to identify issues of medical care, research, and education. Dr. Kenneth I. Shine is president of the Institute of Medicine.

The National Research Council was established by the National Academy of Sciences in 1916 to associate the broad community of science and technology with the Academy's purposes of furthering knowledge and of advising the federal government. Functioning in accordance with general policies determined by the Academy, the Council has become the principal operating agency of both the National Academy of Sciences and the National Academy of Engineering in providing services to the government, the public, and the scientific and engineering communities. The Council is administered jointly by both Academies and the Institute of Medicine. Dr. Bruce Alberts and Dr. William A. Wulf are chairman and vice chairman, respectively, of the National Research Council.

This project was supported by the Department of Transportation under Contract No. DTRS56-98-C-0001. Any opinions, findings, conclusions, or recommendations expressed in this material are those of the authors and do not necessarily express the views of the sponsor.

Available in limited supply from:
National Materials Advisory Board
HA-262
2101 Constitution Avenue, N.W.
Washington, D.C. 20418
202-334-3505
nmab@nas.edu

Additional copies are available for sale from:
National Academy Press
Box 285
2101 Constitution Avenue, N.W.
Washington, D.C. 20055
800-624-6242
202-334-3313 (in the Washington Metropolitan Area)
http://www.nap.edu

International Standard Book Number: 0-309-06776-6
Copyright 1999 by the National Academy of Sciences. All rights reserved.
Printed in the United States of America.

COMMITTEE ON R&D STRATEGIES TO IMPROVE SURFACE TRANSPORTATION SECURITY

H. NORMAN ABRAMSON, *chair*, Southwest Research Institute, San Antonio, Texas
DONALD E. BROWN, University of Virginia, Charlottesville
NICK CARTWRIGHT, Royal Canadian Mounted Police, Ottawa, Ontario, Canada
A. RAY CHAMBERLAIN, Parsons Brinckerhoff, Denver, Colorado
H. ANDY FRANKLIN, Bechtel Technology, Inc., San Francisco, California
ROBERT E. GREEN, JR., Johns Hopkins University, Baltimore, Maryland
BRUCE HADDAN, Norfolk Southern Corporation, Atlanta, Georgia
WILLIAM J. HARRIS, consultant, Arlington, Virginia
MICHAEL L. HONIG, Northwestern University, Evanston, Illinois
JIRI (ART) JANATA, Georgia Institute of Technology, Atlanta
STEVEN B. LIPNER, Mitretek Systems, McLean, Virginia
MICHAEL D. MEYER, Georgia Institute of Technology, Atlanta
FRED V. MORRONE, Port Authority of New York and New Jersey, Jersey City, New Jersey
JULIA WEERTMAN, Northwestern University, Evanston, Illinois

National Research Council Staff

DANIEL MORGAN, study director, senior program officer, National Materials Advisory Board
STEPHEN GODWIN, director, Studies and Information Services, Transportation Research Board
JANE GRIFFITH, interim director, Computer Science and Telecommunications Board
HERB LIN, senior scientist, Computer Science and Telecommunications Board
JANICE PRISCO, senior project assistant, National Materials Advisory Board

NATIONAL MATERIALS ADVISORY BOARD

EDGAR A. STARKE, JR., *chair*, University of Virginia, Charlottesville
JESSE L. (JACK) BEAUCHAMP, California Institute of Technology, Pasadena
EARL H. DOWELL, Duke University, Durham, North Carolina
EDWARD C. DOWLING, Cleveland Cliffs, Inc., Cleveland, Ohio
THOMAS W. EAGAR, Massachusetts Institute of Technology, Cambridge
ALASTAIR M. GLASS, Lucent Technologies, Murray Hill, New Jersey
MARTIN E. GLICKSMAN, Rensselaer Polytechnic Institute, Troy, New York
JOHN A.S. GREEN, The Aluminum Association, Washington, D.C.
SIEGFRIED S. HECKER, Los Alamos National Laboratory, Los Alamos, New Mexico
JOHN H. HOPPS, JR., Morehouse College, Atlanta, Georgia
MICHAEL JAFFE, Rutgers, The State University of New Jersey, New Brunswick
SYLVIA M. JOHNSON, SRI International, Menlo Park, California
SHEILA F. KIA, General Motors Research and Development Center, Warren, Missouri
LISA KLEIN, Rutgers, The State University of New Jersey, New Brunswick
HARRY A. LIPSITT, Wright State University, Dayton, Ohio
ALAN G. MILLER, Boeing Commercial Airplane Group, Seattle, Washington
ROBERT C. PFAHL, JR., Motorola, Schaumburg, Illinois
JULIA M. PHILLIPS, Sandia National Laboratories, Albuquerque, New Mexico
KENNETH L. REIFSNIDER, Virginia Polytechnic Institute and State University, Blacksburg
JAMES W. WAGNER, Case Western Reserve University, Cleveland, Ohio
JULIA R. WEERTMAN, Northwestern University, Evanston, Illinois
BILL G.W. YEE, Pratt & Whitney, West Palm Beach, Florida

RICHARD CHAIT, director

COMPUTER SCIENCE AND TELECOMMUNICATIONS BOARD

DAVID D. CLARK, *chair*, Massachusetts Institute of Technology, Cambridge
FRANCES E. ALLEN, IBM Thomas J. Watson Research Center, Yorktown Heights, New York
JAMES CHIDDIX, Time Warner Cable, Stamford, Connecticut
JOHN M. CIOFFI, Stanford University, Stanford, California
W. BRUCE CROFT, University of Massachusetts, Amherst
A.G. FRASER, AT&T Labs Research, Florham Park, New Jersey
SUSAN L. GRAHAM, University of California, Berkeley
JAMES N. GRAY, Microsoft Corporation, San Francisco, California
PATRICK M. HANRAHAN, Stanford University, Stanford, California
JUDITH HEMPEL, University of California, San Francisco
BUTLER W. LAMPSON, Microsoft Corporation, Cambridge, Massachusetts
EDWARD D. LAZOWSKA, University of Washington, Seattle
DAVID LIDDLE, Interval Research Corporation, Palo Alto, California
JOHN E. MAJOR, WirelessKnowledge, San Diego, California
TOM M. MITCHELL, Carnegie Mellon University, Pittsburgh, Pennsylvania
DONALD NORMAN, Hewlett-Packard, Atherton, California
RAYMOND OZZIE, Groove Networks, Beverly, Massachusetts
DAVID A. PATTERSON, University of California, Berkeley
LEE S. SPROULL, Boston University, Boston, Massachusetts
LESLIE L. VADASZ, Intel Corporation, Santa Clara, California

MARJORY S. BLUMENTHAL, director

TRANSPORTATION RESEARCH BOARD
EXECUTIVE COMMITTEE

WAYNE SHACKELFORD, *chair*, Georgia Department of Transportation, Atlanta
MARTIN WACHS, *vice chair*, University of California, Berkeley
SHARON D. BANKS, AC Transit, Oakland, California
THOMAS F. BARRY, JR., Florida Department of Transportation, Tallahassee
BRIAN J.L. BERRY, University of Texas at Dallas
SARAH C. CAMPBELL, TransManagement, Inc., Washington, D.C.
ANNE P. CANBY, Delaware Department of Transportation, Dover
E. DÈAN CARLSON, Kansas Department of Transportation, Topeka
JOANNE F. CASEY, Intermodal Association of North America, Greenbelt, Maryland
JOHN W. FISHER, Lehigh University, Bethlehem, Pennsylvania
GORMAN GILBERT, North Carolina State University, Raleigh
DELON HAMPTON, Delon Hampton & Associates, Washington, D.C.
LESTER A. HOEL, University of Virginia, Charlottesville
JAMES L. LAMMIE, Parsons Brinckerhoff, Inc., New York, New York
THOMAS F. LARWIN, San Diego Metropolitan Transit Development Board, San Diego, California
BRADLEY L. MALLORY, Pennsylvania Department of Transportation, Harrisburg
JEFFREY J. MCCAIG, Trimac Corporation, Calgary, Alberta, Canada
JOSEPH A. MICKES, Missouri Department of Transportation, Jefferson City
MARSHALL W. MOORE, North Dakota Department of Transportation, Bismarck
JEFFREY R. MORELAND, Burlington Northern Santa Fe Corporation, Fort Worth, Texas
SID MORRISON, Washington State Department of Transportation, Olympia
JOHN P. POORMAN, Capital District Transportation Committee, Albany, New York
ANDREA RINIKER, Port of Tacoma, Tacoma, Washington
JOHN M. SAMUELS, Norfolk Southern Corporation, Norfolk, Virginia
JAMES A. WILDING, Metropolitan Washington Airports Authority, Alexandria, Virginia
CURTIS A. WILEY, Indiana Department of Transportation, Indianapolis
DAVID N. WORMLEY, Pennsylvania State University, University Park

ROBERT E. SKINNER, JR., executive director

Preface

In May 1998, in response to a congressional mandate (House Report 104-863, p. 1189) and with funding from the U.S. Department of Transportation (DOT), the National Research Council formed the Committee on R&D Strategies to Improve Surface Transportation Security. The committee's purpose was to examine the vulnerabilities of the surface transportation system, identify ways to improve the system's security, and recommend a strategy for research and development (R&D). The committee consisted of 14 members with diverse expertise in science, technology, and policy.

The committee was given the following task:

> The study will review the results of the DOT vulnerability assessment to help define areas that could be made less vulnerable with new technologies and processes and which of these technologies and processes are likely to be effective, affordable, and acceptable to the users. This study will identify technologies and processes that hold promise for defending against, mitigating the consequences of, or assisting in the investigation of attacks on the physical surface transportation infrastructure or on the surface transportation information systems and network, including
>
> - technologies and processes in use for other security efforts that may be applied to surface transportation modes with or without modifications
> - technology areas and processes where a development effort or research support may lead to promising surface transportation security technologies
>
> The study will recommend a research and development agenda for the

DOT, including a broad research and development strategy and technology transfer process.

Areas to be addressed include technologies and processes that are specific to an individual transportation mode, as well as those that are crossmodal and intermodal. The study will also consider how these technologies and processes may be effectively transferred to the user communities.

The committee interpreted the word "attacks" primarily to mean attacks by terrorists (or by others using similar methods, such as foreign agents, violent protesters, or disgruntled insiders) rather than conventional criminal activities, such as robberies. Many response strategies might be helpful in both situations, however. In addition, the committee interpreted "attacks on the physical infrastructure" to include human casualties caused by explosions or chemical or biological releases, as well as physical damage, but not to include hijacking or hostage-taking incidents directed primarily at individuals rather than infrastructure. Here too, however, many of the same strategic approaches might be useful in both cases.

Any R&D agenda is based on a set of goals, values, and priorities. During the course of the study, the committee concluded that the first step in establishing an R&D strategy for surface transportation security should be to make that basis explicit. The range of possible security technologies and processes is so broad, the variety of threats so diverse, and the overall security problem so complex that proceeding to the selection of R&D topics without an explicit strategy would give no assurance of an appropriate result.

The committee has not lost sight of the ultimate need to identify specific R&D projects that might improve the security of the surface transportation system. It firmly believes, however, that DOT should put in place a strategy of the type recommended in this report before proceeding to that step. The process of implementing the strategy—such as further evaluating systemic vulnerabilities, establishing a framework for setting priorities, and ensuring the involvement of transportation owners and operators—will elicit essential feedback both from within DOT and from the broader surface transportation community.

This report therefore focuses on the first step, developing a strategic vision of an R&D program for the long term, and recommends a process for achieving that vision. The goal is to present a strategy rather than a shopping list of projects. Several specific R&D topics are discussed, but the report cannot and does not seek to be complete at that level.

The committee met four times between May and November 1998. Meetings included open sessions for gathering information from outside experts, as well as closed deliberative sessions for discussions among the committee members. The third meeting, in August 1998, included a day of site visits to transportation facilities. In addition, selected committee members and staff participated in several outside conferences and workshops during the course of the study to gather information and ideas from the broader transportation and security communities.

Two brief interim letter reports were issued during the course of the study to update DOT on the committee's progress. The present report, the final product of the study, supersedes the two letter reports and presents the committee's complete findings and recommendations.

Acknowledgments

The committee wishes to express its appreciation to the many individuals who provided valuable assistance during the course of the study. The following speakers gave presentations during the first, second, and fourth committee meetings on security and R&D issues in their particular areas of expertise: James Bjostad, Kelley Coyner, John Daly, Mortimer Downey, Thomas Falvey, Jeffrey Shumaker, and Daniel Sullivan, U.S. Department of Transportation; Richard Clarke, National Security Council; John Davis, Critical Infrastructure Assurance Office; Basil Doyle, Federal Bureau of Investigation; Beverly Huey and Richard Little, National Research Council; Kerri-Ann Jones and Steven Rinaldi, Office of Science and Technology Policy; Michael O'Connell and Page Stoutland, U.S. Department of Energy; and Julie Wigton, Counterterrorism Center.

For arranging and hosting the committee's site visits during its third meeting, the committee thanks Beth Brown, Michael Franke, Michael Henry, Ron Hughes, and Hal Whiteman of Transport Canada. Thanks also to those who showed the committee around at the sites: Greg Poitras, Terminal Systems, Inc.; Steve Lefler and Sheena Nelson, BC Ferry Corporation; Fred L. McCague, North West Cruise Ship Association; and K.L. (Kelly) Thomas, VIA Rail Canada.

This study was a joint project of the National Materials Advisory Board of the Commission on Engineering and Technical Systems (CETS), the Computer Science and Telecommunications Board of the Commission on Physical Sciences, Mathematics, and Applications (CPSMA), and the Transportation Research Board (TRB). Joint oversight was provided by a "virtual commission" consisting of James C. Williams, GE Aircraft Engines, and Barry M. Trost, Stanford University, representing CETS; John Kreick, Sanders, a Lockheed Martin Company, and John E. Estes, University of California, Santa Barbara, representing CPSMA; and Lester A. Hoel, University of Virginia, and John M. Samuels, Norfolk Southern Corporation, representing TRB.

This report has been reviewed by individuals chosen for their diverse perspectives and technical expertise, in accordance with procedures approved by the National Research Council's Report Review Committee. The purpose of this independent review is to provide candid and critical comments that will assist the authors and the National Research Council in making their published report as sound as possible and to ensure that the report meets institutional standards for objectivity, evidence, and responsiveness to the study charge. The draft manuscript and the content of the review comments remain confidential to protect the integrity of the deliberative process. The committee wishes to thank the following individuals for their participation in the review of this report: Arden Bement, Purdue University; Trent DePersia, National Institute of Justice; Patrick Griffin, Sandia National Laboratories; Thomas Lambert, Houston Metropolitan Transit Authority; Thomas Larson, consultant; James van Loben Sels, Parsons Brinckerhoff; Fred Schneider, Cornell University; and Joseph Vervier, ENSCO, Inc. While the individuals listed above have provided many constructive comments and suggestions, responsibility for the final content of this report rests solely with the authoring committee and the National Research Council.

Finally, the committee gratefully acknowledges the support of the staff of the National Research Council: Daniel Morgan, Stephen Godwin, Jane Griffith, Herb Lin, and Janice Prisco.

Contents

EXECUTIVE SUMMARY 1

1 INTRODUCTION AND BACKGROUND 3
   The Surface Transportation System, 4
   Federal Security Research and Development, 7
   Characteristics of Surface Transportation Research and Development, 8
   Related Efforts in Infrastructure Protection Policy, 10
   The Organization of This Report, 12

2 ASSESSING VULNERABILITY 13
   Review of the Methodology and Findings of the Department of
     Transportation Vulnerability Assessment, 13
   Assessing Interdependencies and Strategic Vulnerability, 20
   Summary, 27

3 ESTABLISHING A RESEARCH AND DEVELOPMENT
   STRATEGY 28
   Defining the Problem and Objectives, 29
   Identifying Potential Alternatives, 35
   Evaluating Alternatives, 36
   Deciding on a Course of Action, 37
   Implementing the Plan, 37
   Protecting Sensitive Information, 40
   Summary, 42

4   APPLYING THE METHODOLOGY: SOME SPECIFIC RESEARCH
    AND DEVELOPMENT TOPICS 43
    Prevention, 45
    Mitigation, 48
    Monitoring, 53
    Recovery, 56
    Investigation, 57
    Systems Responses, 58
    Summary, 60

5   A VISION OF THE FUTURE 61

REFERENCES 64

APPENDICES
A   Background on Systems Theory 69
B   The Likely Course of Development of Chemical and
    Biological Attacks 71

BIOGRAPHICAL SKETCHES OF COMMITTEE MEMBERS 74

Boxes, Figures, and Tables

BOXES

1-1 Some Incidents Involving Surface Transportation in the United States, 4
1-2 The Sarin Gas Attack on the Tokyo Subway in 1995, 6
1-3 DOT Agencies with R&D Activities, 9

2-1 Nonvirus Cyber Attacks on Surface Transportation, 17
2-2 Differences between Chemical and Biological Attacks, 19
2-3 The Impact of Earthquakes on Surface Transportation, 24
2-4 Implications for Surface Transportation of Trends in Communications, 26

3-1 A Matrix for Categorizing R&D Topics in Surface Transportation Security, 30
3-2 Operators' Perceptions of Threats, 41

4-1 R&D Opportunities in Construction Design, 52

FIGURES

4-1 Platform-edge doors in the London subway, 49

B-1 Flow chart of probable actions in a chemical agent incident, 72
B-2 Flow chart of probable actions in a biological agent incident, 73

TABLES

2-1 Scenarios Considered in the DOT Vulnerability Assessment, 15

4-1 Illustration of the Matrix Categorization of R&D Topics, 44

Executive Summary

The surface transportation system is vital to our nation's economy, defense, and quality of life. Because threats against the system have hitherto been perceived as minor, little attention has been paid to its security. But the world is changing, as highlighted by dramatic incidents such as the terrorist chemical attack on the Tokyo subway in 1995. As a consequence, security concerns are now attracting more attention—appropriately so, for the threat is real, and responding to it is hard. Although the surface transportation system is remarkably resilient, it is also open and decentralized, making a security response challenging. Research and development can contribute to that response in important ways.

The first step is to develop a better understanding of the problem. The U.S. Department of Transportation (DOT) has already begun this effort by assessing the surface transportation system's vulnerability to hostile attacks. The present study finds that assessment to be a valuable and commendable foundation. Further work is needed in some areas, particularly regarding chemical, biological, and cyber attacks, and especially the strategic vulnerability of the surface transportation system as a whole that may result from internal and external interdependencies.

All aspects of this problem are still new and relatively ill defined in comparison with other, more established fields, such as aviation security. DOT must continue its efforts to improve its understanding of the problem. The assessment of vulnerabilities should be ongoing and should be expanded to include systemic vulnerabilities beyond local damage and disruption. Intelligence efforts to identify likely threats should continue. An analysis of past incidents, including natural disasters and major accidents, which have many similarities with intentional attacks, should seek to identify both best practices and areas of technology need. Research and development must always be recognized as part of this broader picture.

DOT's first priority in setting up a research and development program for the security of surface transportation should be to define and put in place a clear and comprehensive strategy. That strategy should be founded on a systematic process of five steps: clear definition of the problem and objectives, identification of a wide variety of possible solutions, rigorous evaluation of those alternatives, careful decision making, and effective implementation. This process should be implemented across transportation modes, rather than separately for each mode. It should be coordinated proactively with other agencies, and DOT should understand and clearly delineate the boundaries of its role relative to those agencies. A variety of stakeholders from inside and outside the government should be involved closely, through mechanisms such as workshops to help evaluate proposed activities. As the effort grows, DOT will increasingly need a way to protect information that is sensitive but not classified. Finally, and perhaps most important, the strategy must recognize the vital importance of involving the owners and operators of surface transportation, whose participation in the process and acceptance of its objectives will ultimately determine whether the results are actually implemented and security is actually improved.

Some important themes emerge from analysis of this strategy. First, a dual-use approach, in which security objectives are furthered at the same time as other transportation goals, can encourage the implementation of security technologies and processes. Second, modeling could be used more to develop a better understanding of the scope of the security problem. Third, DOT can play an important role in developing and disseminating information about best practices that use existing technologies and processes, including low-technology alternatives. Finally, security should be considered as part of a broader picture, not a wholly new and different problem but one that is similar and closely connected to the transportation community's previous experience in responding to accidents, natural disasters, and hazardous materials.

Specific findings and recommendations are summarized at the end of each chapter and are presented for reference in Chapter 5.

1

Introduction and Background

Surface transportation in the United States is an extraordinarily large and complex system responsible for the movement of vast numbers of passengers and vast quantities of freight via road, rail, water, and pipeline. The system includes many thousands of independent, interlocking operators, some small and some large, some public and some private. The system's efficiency and convenience are essential to the strength of our economy, the security of our nation, and the quality of our lives.

For a variety of reasons, security against hostile attacks is rarely a high priority for surface transportation. This situation is unlike the case of aviation, for which a series of incidents in the late 1960s and early 1970s inspired an extensive program of technological and procedural security measures (NRC, 1999). Yet because of the surface transportation system's importance and vulnerability, as highlighted by several recent studies and high-profile incidents, improving security is essential. This study considers research and development (R&D) strategies to improve the security of all modes of surface transportation (but not aviation) against such threats as bombings, intentional chemical and biological releases, and cyber attacks. (See Box 1-1 for some examples of recent incidents.)

Numerous federal agencies conduct R&D on security measures against hostile attacks. Much of that work is generally applicable. Work in related areas, particularly protection against natural disasters and accidents, is also relevant. Interagency information sharing and coordination are thus extremely important elements of any security R&D effort. Capitalizing on these broader efforts while

> **BOX 1-1**
> **Some Incidents Involving Surface Transportation in the United States**
>
> 1977   Bombs explode on a Florida highway to protest the Panama Canal Treaty
> 1980   Pipe bombs placed by a Puerto Rican nationalist group explode in Penn Station lockers
> 1982   Liquid explosive found in a car parked under the Bay Bridge in San Francisco
> 1984   Bomb threat on a Florida bridge
> 1986   Bomb threat on a Massachusetts bridge in support of striking fishermen
> 1987   Bomb threat on a Missouri bridge
> 1992   Hand grenade found in a Chicago commuter rail station
> 1993   Muslim fundamentalists arrested in a plot to blow up tunnels and a bridge in New York
> 1993   Bomb threat on bridges near Niagara Falls
> 1994   Bombs explode in the New York subway (two incidents) to extort money from the city
> 1995   Train intentionally derailed in Arizona probably by right-wing extremists or a former railroad employee
> 1995   New York subway token booth set on fire
>
> Source: Mineta Institute, 1997.

identifying the unique role of the U.S. Department of Transportation (DOT) is a key challenge.

Now that the Cold War is over, security concerns in many fields are being focused increasingly on the threat of terrorism, whether by an organized state or state-sponsored group as a form of "asymmetrical warfare" or by a nonstate group or individual motivated by extremist ideology or hatred. The present study is just one of many recent and continuing efforts to address this problem, either in broad terms or with a specific focus on individual sectors of the nation's infrastructure.

The goal of this chapter is to provide an overview of these issues as background for the remainder of the report. The chapter concludes with a brief description of the general structure and approach of the report.

THE SURFACE TRANSPORTATION SYSTEM

The U.S. surface transportation system is large, complex, and decentralized. DOT, despite its regulatory and other responsibilities for transportation, actually owns or operates almost none of the system. This makes addressing surface transportation security concerns particularly challenging. In particular, it means that any R&D program at DOT must pay special attention to the process of transferring technology to owners and operators.

Another consequence of the decentralized nature of surface transportation is its resiliency in responding to disruptions, whether caused by intentional attacks, accidents, or natural disasters. Except in a few major metropolitan areas, and except during peak periods even in those areas, the system usually has redundant capacity—alternate routes and alternate transportation modes. Although even a single attack could cause significant destruction and distress, as well as reduce public confidence in the transportation system, it is hard to imagine a single attack that could shut down a large city, let alone a region or the country as a whole. Multiple, coordinated attacks or attacks that directly affect a wide area— such as attacks on control or communications systems, particularly as surface transportation becomes increasingly computerized and automated—raise different concerns. And redundancy is low in some specific cases, such as passenger transport in major cities during peak commuting periods, or some types of freight transport.

The goal of the transportation system is to be open, accessible, free flowing, and convenient. Many security measures are inherently restrictive and hence run counter to this goal. For example, it is hard to imagine instituting airport-style security checkpoints on highways. Thus the system's openness and accessibility sometimes make it more vulnerable.

Moreover, because transportation systems bring masses of people together and are highly visible and familiar, they are particularly attractive targets. In 1996, there were at least 631 violent attacks against surface transportation worldwide (DOT, 1998b). Most attacks are bombings, but the targets and incidents vary widely and include such well known cases as the hijacking of the *Achille Lauro* cruise ship in 1985 and the sarin gas attack on the Tokyo subway in 1995 (see Box 1-2). So far, the U.S. transportation system has experienced very few incidents. Nevertheless, the attacks that have occurred (along with several high-profile attacks against other U.S. targets, such as the bombing of a federal office building in Oklahoma City in 1995 and the bombings of U.S. embassies overseas in 1998) and high-profile attacks against transportation in other countries have raised the level of concern considerably. Because threats change over time as the world situation changes and as security is tightened in other areas, DOT and others should be proactive in preparing for the future despite the low frequency of recent attacks on surface transportation in the United States. The responsible agencies would be most unwise to wait passively until a major incident brings calls for action which they would then be ill prepared to meet.

Finally, the huge impact of even unintentional breakdowns, when they do occur despite the system's usual resiliency, makes clear the enormous potential consequences of intentional attacks against surface transportation. For example,

BOX 1-2
The Sarin Gas Attack on the Tokyo Subway in 1995

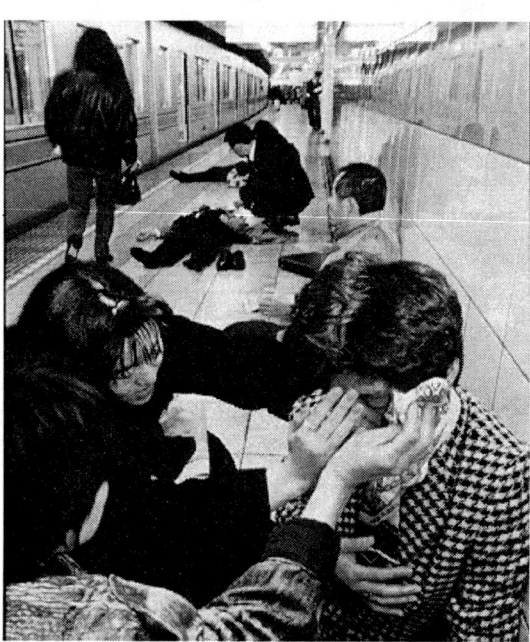

Victims receive assistance on a Tokyo subway platform. Source unknown.

During rush hour on a Monday morning in March 1995, a Japanese cult released the nerve agent sarin in the Tokyo subway. Even tiny quantities of this chemical are deadly. The sarin was concealed in lunch boxes and soft-drink containers, placed on train floors, and released by puncturing the containers with umbrellas as the terrorists left the trains.

Firefighters were the first emergency personnel to arrive on the scene. They were not equipped with any antidote, and even if they had been, they had no idea what substance they were dealing with.

Many victims made their own way to hospitals by car or taxi. The treatment of arriving casualties varied from hospital to hospital. At one, staff members were unaware of the nature of the incident for several hours and so made no attempt at decontamination. As a result, more than 20 percent of the staff who treated victims at that hospital developed symptoms themselves. At another hospital, staff initially believed they were dealing with cyanide poisoning.

By noon the next day 5,510 patients had reported to medical facilities. Eight died on the first day and four more in the following month.

Sources: Ohbu et al., 1997; Neifert, 1996.

in Texas alone, service disruptions following a major railroad merger in 1996 are estimated to have cost shippers at least $1 billion in delays, lost production and sales, and higher shipping costs (Weinstein and Clower, 1998). In a system this vast, a loss of public confidence, even in the absence of actual attacks, could have a significant economic impact.

FEDERAL SECURITY RESEARCH AND DEVELOPMENT

A variety of U.S. federal agencies conduct security-related R&D; most of them are not directly concerned with surface transportation. They include the agencies and services of the Department of Defense (at numerous laboratories and covering a broad range of topics), the Department of Energy and its national laboratories (also very broad), the Department of Justice (focused primarily on tools for law enforcement personnel), the Federal Aviation Administration (focused on bomb and weapon attacks against aircraft), the Department of Health and Human Services (focused on biological and chemical attacks), the Department of Commerce (including work on cyber security at the National Institute of Standards and Technology), the Central Intelligence Agency, the Department of the Treasury, the Department of State, and others. This diversity is significant for DOT's role in security R&D in two ways: interagency coordination and information sharing are critical, and DOT's own efforts must be focused sharply on areas where it is the agency best placed to make effective progress.

Coordination and information sharing are a major challenge for DOT and, indeed, for all agencies involved in addressing security issues.[1] The most basic problem is just finding out what work is being done. For DOT to capitalize on the results of R&D by other agencies and work effectively with them, it will have to make strenuous efforts to acquire a clearer picture of the situation than is currently available. To that end, DOT should continue its active and long-term participation in such coordinating organizations as the Critical Infrastructure Coordinating Group's interagency working group on R&D (supported by the Critical Infrastructure Assurance Office) and the Technical Support Working Group (an interagency activity led by the Departments of Defense, State, and Energy).

Because security is a concern that cuts across agency boundaries, another challenge for DOT will be to identify its appropriate role in the overall security R&D effort. That role will be vitally important, but in an overall picture that

---

[1] This challenge is not new or unique to DOT. A 1997 General Accounting Office report that considered all federal agencies found that federal funding for "programs and activities to combat terrorism is unknown and difficult to determine." The same report found "no basis to have reasonable assurance" that policy and strategy are coordinated and focused, that activities and capabilities are "not unnecessarily duplicative or redundant," or that "funding gaps or misallocations have not occurred" (GAO, 1997).

includes such R&D giants as the Department of Defense and the Department of Energy, it will also be relatively small. DOT should therefore focus its efforts sharply on meeting the specific needs of surface transportation. Probably DOT's main emphasis will be on the adaptation, synthesis, implementation, and deployment of existing or low-technology solutions and on the development and dissemination of best practices for transportation owners and operators, rather than on long-term basic research or the development of new high-technology hardware or software.

CHARACTERISTICS OF SURFACE TRANSPORTATION RESEARCH AND DEVELOPMENT

A brief overview of the character and structure of surface transportation R&D in general may provide a useful perspective on the context for specifically security-related R&D. DOT is the single largest source of R&D funding for nondefense surface transportation. Although its share is less than a quarter of the total, it acts as a catalyst for other funders, which include state and local governments and the private sector. These other groups are particularly important in ensuring that R&D results are implemented. The remainder of this section focuses on DOT because security-related transportation R&D is likely to receive most support at the federal level, but the roles of others, particularly in implementation, should not be neglected.

DOT is made up of several agencies, most of them defined by particular transportation modes. Their R&D efforts (see Box 1-3) are not centralized, although the Office of the Secretary, which includes an Office of Intelligence and Security, provides coordination and strategic planning. This dispersed structure has significant implications for R&D in crosscutting areas such as security.

R&D is not the primary focus of any DOT agency. For the most part, DOT agencies are focused on regulatory functions and on the transfer of federal transportation funding to state and local agencies. For example, as shown in Box 1-3, about three-quarters of DOT's surface transportation R&D is funded by the Federal Highway Administration (FHWA); nevertheless, R&D accounts for only 1.7 percent of FHWA's total budget. For the department as a whole, R&D accounts for only 1.8 percent of total expenditures.

Because DOT agencies have specific missions, the R&D they support tends to focus on applied topics that are narrowly defined. Projects are usually directed toward specific deliverables, rather than being open-ended or exploratory. Very little basic research is supported. Funds are typically awarded via contracts rather than grants or cooperative agreements, and although these contracts are usually awarded competitively, the proposals are usually reviewed by agency staff rather than peer researchers. A large fraction of R&D funding is congressionally directed ("earmarked") for specific institutions or activities. Together, the applied, mission-specific focus of most programs and the prevalence of detailed

BOX 1-3
DOT Agencies with R&D Activities

DOT Agency	FY99 Funding R&D (in M$)	FY99 Funding Total (in M$)	R&D (%)	Major R&D Areas
Federal Highway Administration	462	27,367	1.7	construction materials and processes, safety, environment, data gathering and policy analysis, intelligent transportation systems
National Highway Traffic Safety Administration	72	360	20.0	biomechanics, crash avoidance, vehicle safety systems, data collection and analysis, driver behavior
Federal Transit Administration	58	5,388	1.1	access for the disabled, air quality, traffic congestion, safety, innovative vehicles, regional planning
Federal Railroad Administration	43	778	5.5	safety, high-speed rail, magnetically levitated trains
U.S. Coast Guard	17	4,302	0.4	mission-related technologies, materials, and human factors
Office of the Secretary	9	87	10.3	policy analysis, systems development
Research and Special Programs Administration[a]	7	72	9.7	planning, assessment, pipeline safety, transportation of hazardous materials
Federal Aviation Administration	226	9,754	2.3	aircraft structures and materials, aviation security
Other[b]	0	242	0.0	
Total	894	48,351	1.8	

[a] The Research and Special Programs Administration operates the John A. Volpe National Transportation Systems Center, which conducts R&D under contract for other DOT and non-DOT agencies. To prevent double counting, this contract funding is not shown separately in the table. Typically it amounts to about $200 million per year.

[b] Includes Bureau of Transportation Statistics, Saint Lawrence Seaway Development Corporation, Maritime Administration, Office of the Inspector General, and Surface Transportation Board.

Note: The figures given here are totals for "Research, Development, and Technology." For most agencies, these are the sums of subtotals for "R&D," "Technology," and "Facilities." There are many ways to define R&D and the types of activity it includes. The purpose of this table is to give a general sense of the scope of DOT's R&D activities in surface transportation. The committee has not attempted either to reconcile the definitions used by different sources or to judge the appropriateness of definitions.

Source: DOT, 1999a, 1999b.

congressional direction severely limit DOT's discretion to increase support for security-related R&D using existing funds.

The main opportunity for investigator-initiated R&D is through the University Transportation Centers program, which provides about $32 million per year in matching funds for research, education, and technology transfer. None of the centers currently specializes in security-related topics.

RELATED EFFORTS IN INFRASTRUCTURE PROTECTION POLICY

Efforts to protect the surface transportation system are only a small part of recent efforts throughout the federal government to protect critical national infrastructures. These efforts include two presidential decision directives, the work of the Presidential Commission on Critical Infrastructure Protection (PCCIP) and its successor the Critical Infrastructure Assurance Office, and DOT's own efforts at vulnerability assessment. A brief overview of these activities may help to place surface transportation issues in context.

The PCCIP was formed by executive order in July 1996 and consisted of 18 senior representatives from private industry, government, and academia. It was charged with identifying critical infrastructures, assessing their vulnerabilities, and formulating a comprehensive national strategy for protecting them from physical and cyber threats. An infrastructure was considered critical if its incapacity or destruction would have a debilitating effect on the defense or economic security of the nation. The PCCIP determined that the critical infrastructures are transportation, telecommunications, electrical power, gas and oil distribution, banking and finance, water supply, government services, and emergency services. It concluded that the threat is real, the vulnerabilities are extensive, and the responsibility for addressing the problem should be shared by the government and private-sector owners and operators. Among the wide range of actions the PCCIP recommended in its final report was an increase in R&D (PCCIP, 1997).

The President subsequently issued two presidential decision directives. *Combating Terrorism* (PDD-62) lays out a new and more systematic management approach for federal counterterrorism activities. Its key element is the identification of organizational responsibilities of federal agencies. In addition, it establishes the position of national coordinator for security, infrastructure protection, and counterterrorism at the National Security Council. The coordinator is responsible for overseeing policies and programs in counterterrorism, protection of critical infrastructures, preparedness, and consequence management.

Critical Infrastructure Protection (PDD-63) sets out a program of federal actions to improve the security of critical infrastructures. These include identifying and assessing vulnerabilities, planning to reduce exposure to attack, and improving cooperation between the government and the private sector. In each infrastructure area, including transportation, a federal liaison official and a private-sector coordinator will work together. (For transportation, the National Defense Transportation Association is expected to serve as private-sector coordinator.) Achieving private-sector buy-in is generally seen as the most significant challenge for the implementation of PDD-63. The goal is to achieve an initial operating capability for protection of critical infrastructures by 2000 and a full operating capability by 2003.

The Critical Infrastructure Assurance Office, which is housed in the Department of Commerce, was formed in May 1998 as a result of PDD-63. It has several responsibilities:

- integration of plans for individual sectors into a national infrastructure assurance plan
- coordination of analysis of the federal government's dependencies on critical infrastructures
- coordination of national education and awareness efforts and other public and legislative activities related to infrastructure protection
- support of the national coordinator for security, infrastructure protection, and counterterrorism, the interagency Critical Infrastructure Coordinating Group, and the National Infrastructure Assurance Council

In July 1998, the Critical Infrastructure Assurance Office published the report of a multiagency road-mapping effort for infrastructure protection R&D (CIAO, 1998). Coordinated by a group from Argonne National Laboratory, this effort involved a large team from a variety of federal and private-sector organizations. The group examined the critical infrastructure sectors identified in the PCCIP report as a first step in "developing a robust and harmonized national research and development plan that comprehensively addresses critical infrastructure assurance needs" (p. vii). The discussion of the transportation sector discussed four categories of R&D topics:

- identification and measurement of and awareness training for system vulnerabilities
- development and adaptation of monitoring, detection, mitigation, and incident response hardware
- development and adaptation of monitoring, detection, mitigation, and incident response software
- information assurance, human factors, and institutional effects in preparedness and response

The primary focus was on cyber attacks; the threat of physical attacks was less prominent; chemical and biological threats were mostly left to others to address (Davis, 1998).

THE ORGANIZATION OF THIS REPORT

The remainder of this report is structured as follows. Chapter 2 presents the study's evaluation of DOT's vulnerability assessment for surface transportation and recommends some ways to improve on it in future assessments. The recommendations give particular attention to the important and underrecognized question of strategic vulnerabilities, that is, vulnerabilities of the surface transportation infrastructure as a whole as distinct from vulnerabilities of individual infrastructure elements. Chapter 3 discusses a systematic approach to establishing an R&D strategy. It focuses on the process of planning a program (defining, selecting, and evaluating potential R&D projects) rather than on the details of specific projects. Because threats to the surface transportation infrastructure are constantly evolving, careful attention to this planning process will be vital for keeping the program on target. Finally, Chapter 4 attempts a preliminary application of the methodology recommended in Chapter 3, and in doing so, presents some examples of the kinds of R&D projects that might be considered.

Note that this study has intentionally not divided up its subject according to the various modes of transportation. Although most transportation-related R&D is funded and organized according to mode, there is so much synergy and overlap among the security concerns of the different modes that such a division in this report would be artificial and even deleterious. An important conclusion of the study is the need for close coordination and cooperation, not only within DOT, but also with other agencies. Emphasizing the differences between the transportation modes would make that coordination more difficult.

2

Assessing Vulnerability

The starting point of the study that produced this report was a vulnerability assessment prepared by DOT (1998a). The committee's first task was to review that assessment as a foundation for defining areas that new technologies and processes could make less vulnerable and for identifying which of those technologies and processes might be effective, affordable, and acceptable to users. This chapter presents key elements of the committee's review.[1] It also addresses the important question of strategic vulnerabilities, that is, the effect of attacks on the transportation system as a whole, beyond their effect on any individual targeted element of the system.

REVIEW OF THE METHODOLOGY AND FINDINGS OF THE DEPARTMENT OF TRANSPORTATION VULNERABILITY ASSESSMENT

Overall, the DOT vulnerability assessment is excellent, and DOT is to be commended for producing a useful report. The assessment clearly demonstrates the validity of concerns about security in surface transportation and lays a good foundation for addressing those concerns via an R&D program.

---

[1] Many of these points were made in previous communications from the committee to DOT (which are superceded by this report). The committee understands that DOT is revising the vulnerability assessment in response to those communications.

General Methodology

The DOT vulnerability assessment explicitly avoids assessing the probability of any given type of attack occurring. Instead, it examines a variety of scenarios for possible attacks and assesses the damage that could be caused in each scenario, including both human casualties and economic losses. A key finding of the assessment is a categorization of each scenario as to the likelihood of success if the attack were attempted and the resulting impact if the attack succeeded. The likelihood of success is rated as improbable, moderately probable, highly probable, or certain. The potential impact is rated as not serious, moderately serious, very serious, or catastrophic.

The assessment process used a nine-step methodology:

1. *Identification of assets*, such as facilities, vehicles, and equipment, based on the expert knowledge of DOT and industry personnel
2. S*creening of the criticality of assets* and selection of key assets for further evaluation based on the high impact their loss would have (as determined by expert opinion) on people or system operations or both
3. *Identification of threats to critical assets* based on historical data and expert opinion;
4. *Formulation of scenarios* by pairing the critical assets identified in Step 2 with the threats identified in Step 3
5. *Assessment of the vulnerability of assets in each scenario*, i.e., assessment of the characteristics (such as ease of access or presence of security measures) that make an asset easy or difficult to attack
6. *Assessment of the impact of an attack in each scenario*, focusing on deaths, injuries, property damage, and loss of service
7. *Categorization of scenarios by likelihood of loss and severity of impact*
8. *Review of consistency* by a panel of experts to ensure that scenarios involving different modes of transportation were assessed on comparable scales
9. *Identification of potential countermeasures*

DOT acknowledges that the scenarios are illustrative, not exhaustive, but they cover a wide range of possible targets and attacks (see Table 2-1).

The vulnerability assessment states clearly that it analyzes only the vulnerabilities of surface transportation assets, without regard to the likelihood of any particular threat. (Presumably, though, the threats identified in Step 3 above are considered at least plausible. Just selecting scenarios for consideration implicitly constitutes a first-order assessment of their likelihood.) The methodology used is appropriate and adequate for such an analysis, and for the most part, the selection of scenarios is comprehensive and illustrates the methodology well. In addition

TABLE 2-1 Scenarios Considered in the DOT Vulnerability Assessment

Physical Attacks
- car bomb at bridge approach
- series of small explosives on highway bridge
- single small explosive on highway bridge
- single small explosive in highway tunnel
- car bomb in highway tunnel
- series of car bombs on adjacent bridges or tunnels
- bomb(s) detonated at pipeline compressor stations
- bomb detonated at pipeline storage facility
- bomb detonated on pipeline segment
- simultaneous attacks on ports
- terrorist bombing of waterfront pavilion
- container vessel fire at marine terminal
- ramming of railroad bridge by maritime vessel
- attack on passenger vessel in port
- shooting in rail station
- vehicle bomb adjacent to rail station
- bombing of airport transit station
- bombing of underwater transit tunnel
- bus bombing
- deliberate blocking of highway-rail grade crossing
- terrorist bombing of rail tunnel
- bomb detonated on train in rail station
- vandalism of track structure and signal system
- terrorist bombing of rail bridge
- explosives attack on multiple rail bridges
- explosive in cargo of passenger aircraft

Biological Attacks
- biological release in highway tunnel
- anthrax release from freight ship
- anthrax release in transit station
- anthrax release on passenger train

Chemical Attacks
- sarin release in multiple subway stations
- physical attack on railcar carrying a toxic chemical

Cyber and C^3 Attacks
- cyber attack on highway traffic control system
- cyber attack on pipeline automated control system
- attack on port power and telecommunications facility
- sabotage of train control system
- tampering with rail signals
- cyber attack on train control center

to the review of consistency that was conducted by an expert panel (Step 8), the basic assumptions and predicted consequences of each scenario should be subjected to a further reality check, in cooperation with representatives of the relevant transportation industries. (The present study does not attempt to examine individual scenarios at this level of detail. Doing so would require input from a much larger, broader group.)

Threat Analysis

In order to develop an appropriate response strategy consisting of policy changes or a program of R&D, further analysis of the likelihood of different threats is highly desirable. The DOT assessment identified threats based on input from a combination of historical data, surveys, and the advice of security experts, but its goal was to assess vulnerabilities, not risks or threats. A threat analysis would require much more detailed consideration of these inputs. It would also, of course, make the resulting report a much more sensitive document. Moreover, the committee recognizes the great difficulty of such an analysis, including the limitations of extrapolating from historical data as the methods and targets of attackers continue to evolve. This question is revisited briefly in Chapter 3 in the discussion of setting priorities for R&D.

Means of Attack

The vulnerability assessment includes a nine-page chapter on possible means of attack against surface transportation. Such a brief discussion is appropriate as background for the vulnerability assessment, but future efforts to extend the assessment will have to be based on a more complete, balanced, and clearly defined analysis of the various means of threat delivery.

Cyber and C^3 Attacks

Cyber attacks and other attacks on the command, control, and communications (C^3) systems of surface transportation are not given enough attention or analysis in the assessment. This lack of emphasis may have been an attempt to avoid duplicating other ongoing efforts, such as the work of the PCCIP. Nevertheless, the transportation industries' increasing use of automation and telecommunications makes consideration of cyber and C^3 attacks essential, especially the interrelationships among cyber attacks and noncyber attacks directed against C^3 targets. Discussion of the transportation sector's use of the Global Positioning System (GPS) is also lacking. The need to examine cyber and C^3 vulnerabilities is part of the broader need to examine systemic, or strategic, interdependencies and vulnerabilities.

The discussion of cyber attacks that does appear in the DOT assessment focuses mostly on the introduction of computer viruses into computer-based control centers and the resulting disruption or denial of automated services. Unfortunately, one can easily envision scenarios with much more destructive effects (Box 2-1).

As this report was nearing completion, an outbreak of the Melissa computer virus drew considerable media attention. Implemented as a computer program

---

BOX 2-1
Nonvirus Cyber Attacks on Surface Transportation

Not all cyber attacks involve computer viruses. Moreover, other types of cyber attack can sometimes be more damaging. For example, vulnerabilities may be created if intelligent transportation system (ITS) control centers are linked to the Internet so that travelers can assess traffic levels and delays before departing on their journeys. An attacker could exploit an improperly configured traffic information web server to modify and execute programs known as CGI scripts. The ability to execute such programs would allow an attacker to take control of the web server. From there, an attacker would have to penetrate a firewall to get to the network where the ITS control system computers reside. If that firewall were improperly configured, and if the attacker could gain access to CGI scripts or other programs on a computer on the control system network, he or she would probably be able to disrupt or modify the ITS real-time control computers. Because these computers are protected by the firewall and used for real-time applications, they are likely to be configured with little or no security. The attacker's choices would then range from crashing the control system, which would simply be disruptive, to changing control parameters, programs, or data, which might cause a system-wide incident and result in delays or loss of life. Achieving maximum impact would require considerable knowledge about the ITS control system, of course, which could probably only be gained by exhaustively and painstakingly reviewing purloined data and programs or by exploiting the expertise of a current or former control center programmer or operator.

Another way to attack an ITS system would be to modify the control software during development. Software developers and development systems are often not as well protected as operational systems. Moreover, the presence in the development environment of programming source code (and probably documentation regarding requirements and designs) makes it easier to design an attack. The attack software would have to pass the developer's quality assurance and configuration management systems, but methods for embedding hostile software that does not appear in source code listings and is not detectable by functional testing have long been known in the computer science community (see Thompson, 1984). The usual process of software distribution would then distribute the attack to all sites that used the ITS software.

As these and other examples show, the vulnerability of the surface transportation system to cyber attacks is a real concern, and DOT should take it very seriously.

embedded in a word processor document, Melissa spread copies of itself automatically via e-mail when the document was read. This caused network congestion and user confusion, but like most virus incidents, it was apparently not intended to destroy or disclose sensitive information. The Melissa experience is instructive, however, because another attacker might use a similar mechanism to propagate a more targeted, more hostile code with the aim of damaging a particular user or system. For example, such a mechanism might be used to attack an ITS control center or an ITS software development site.

Chemical and Biological Attacks

In scenarios involving chemical and biological attacks, future assessments should make more careful distinctions between the consequences of chemical attacks and biological attacks and between the consequences of attacks involving various agents with different properties.

Although chemical and biological attacks are often considered together—the phrase "chem/bio" is sometimes used almost as a single word—they are in fact different in many ways, particularly as a consequence of the incubation period associated with biological agents (see Box 2-2 and Appendix B).[2] For example, the "first responders" after a biological attack are likely to be hospital staff or public health officials, not police, fire, or emergency medical personnel at the scene of an incident. Unless real-time biological detection systems are developed and deployed (which seems highly unlikely for the foreseeable future), a biological attack may not even be noticed until well after it has taken place.

It is also important to consider differences between the physical and chemical properties of different agents, such as density, phase, toxicity, and speed of action. The DOT assessment includes just two scenarios for chemical attacks, a release of the liquid nerve agent sarin as an aerosol and a release of a toxic industrial gas. Of the four biological scenarios, three involve anthrax and one does not specify the agent. Attacks with other agents could have quite different characteristics and implications with regard to the dispersion of the agent and other factors. A wider variety of scenarios should be considered, therefore, including agents that may not be suitable for military use. Some military requirements, such as mass production, weaponization, and safe storage, may not apply to nonmilitary attackers. Thus chemical and biological terrorism are not necessarily the same as chemical and biological warfare. For example, a variety of dangerous

---

[2] The "most basic" general conclusion of a recent study was that "terrorist incidents involving biological agents, especially infectious agents, are likely to be very different from those involving chemical agents and thus demand very different preparation and response (the myriad of 'chemical/biological' response teams being developed at federal, state, and local levels are, in fact, almost entirely focused on detection, decontamination, and expedient treatment of chemical casualties)" (IOM and NRC, 1999).

> **BOX 2-2**
> **Differences between Chemical and Biological Attacks**
>
> It is a serious misapprehension to assume that chemical and biological attacks are similar. Here are some of the important differences:
> - A *chemical* attack disperses a highly toxic chemical (which may be either synthetic or biological in origin) that acts rapidly on the target. Symptoms become evident after only a short time. The release site can be easily and quickly identified. Emergency personnel at the scene are the first responders. Decontamination is usually critical, but once victims have been decontaminated, they need not be kept in isolation.
> - A *biological* attack delivers living organisms, such as bacteria or viruses, that require an incubation period, often days or even weeks, to reach full potency. Identifying the time and location of the release may be extremely difficult. Medical and public health personnel throughout the community are the "first responders." No decontamination is necessary, but in many cases, isolating victims is essential to prevent the spread of the disease.
>
> Source: Henderson, 1999.

chemicals are easily available from sources such as hardware and farm supply stores. These chemicals do not have the military-grade toxicity of sarin, but they are still highly toxic.

Finally, chemical and biological vulnerabilities should be considered carefully and seriously and not left to others to worry about.

The Need for a Continuing Effort

The DOT vulnerability assessment, although very valuable to the transportation industry and others, should not be a one-time effort. Rather, it should be the first installment in a continuing series of analyses. The same is true of the analysis of R&D strategies that this report seeks to initiate. Future assessments should draw on the wide variety of techniques used by other public and private organizations to evaluate and manage threats and risks and protect assets and operations. For example, just as computer security companies sometimes have a staff of "red team" hackers, DOT might establish a working group (or participate actively in one with broader sponsorship) in which some participants play the role of attackers and others seek improved defenses. At a minimum, this would improve DOT's understanding of best practices in the use of existing security technologies and processes.

Sensitive Information

A final concern, which the committee shares with DOT and others, is the potential that this type of assessment could be misused by groups or individuals with hostile intentions. It is unfortunate that current guidelines for the protection of sensitive information provide no solution to this problem. This topic is discussed further in Chapter 3.

ASSESSING INTERDEPENDENCIES AND STRATEGIC VULNERABILITY

A recurring theme of discussion during the course of this study was the distinction between attacks against a single element of the surface transportation infrastructure (point attacks) and attacks against the infrastructure as a whole (systemic attacks). The diverse elements of the surface transportation system are often highly interdependent; for example, disabling a major urban subway system during rush hour could cause an overflow of travelers onto local roads and highways that are already extremely crowded. The growing use of information technology in command and control systems for surface transportation is introducing new interdependencies. Transportation is highly interdependent with other infrastructure sectors, too, such as the power grid and the telecommunications network. Finally, attacks against certain critical nodes, such as a port that might be the single planned point of departure for military units during an international crisis, could have an impact far beyond the impact of a similar attack on an otherwise similar target. These strategic vulnerabilities, and ways to respond to them, are the subject of the remainder of this chapter. They were not considered in any depth in the DOT vulnerability assessment, but they warrant close attention.

Interdependencies in the Surface Transportation System

Because of the decentralized, multimodal character of surface transportation, mounting a system-wide attack with large spatial and temporal impact would be difficult. Experience with natural disasters suggests that even the simultaneous destruction of multiple elements of the system has less impact on its ability to operate than one might expect. The surface transportation infrastructure has many redundancies and is quite resilient. In most places, at most times, a variety of transportation options and alternate routes are available. Moreover, although multiple, coordinated attacks could have systemic consequences, the logistical difficulty of coordinating them would increase both the required expertise and the likelihood of detection or prevention.

Nevertheless, in order to understand surface transportation's systemic vulnerabilities better, DOT should undertake a study of the system's redundancies. The study should identify interdependencies and redundancies among the components of the surface transportation system and critical nodes (perhaps major bridges, pipelines, harbors, or transit interchanges) where a lack of redundancy creates systemic vulnerability. Besides identifying areas of vulnerability, the results would probably provide useful insights into ways of taking advantage of redundancies when seeking to recover smoothly from a point attack. This type of study, focused on strategic vulnerabilities rather than tactical vulnerabilities (as in the work DOT has undertaken so far), might require simulation or "wargaming" exercises.

Interdependencies and Cyber Attacks

The growing and evolving automation of the transportation infrastructure, particularly the introduction of infrastructure-wide automation systems, may increase the opportunities for infrastructure-wide attacks. Such attacks could interfere with routing or resource allocation mechanisms or cause physical damage to infrastructure elements across a wide area.

Most computer and network systems have a variety of software vulnerabilities, and attackers have developed many techniques for exploiting them to gain control of individual computers or entire networks. It is extremely difficult to build a complex piece of software that not only performs its intended function but also is invulnerable to malicious abuse. For example, despite the widespread attention given to the 1988 Internet Worm, a highly publicized attack on the program that routes electronic mail from computer to computer across the Internet, attacks on the same program continue to be reported. The computers and networks that control and monitor transportation systems are no exception to this general situation in their vulnerability to cyber attacks.

A malicious and effective attack against a network or infrastructure, however, could be far more serious than the attacks by hackers that are so often reported in the popular and trade press. Hackers regularly demonstrate their ability to take control of systems and crash them or destroy data. Security products are commercially available that, when properly configured, can defeat many such attacks, even by relatively sophisticated and hostile hackers. A sufficiently sophisticated attacker may still have a reasonable chance of success, however, and in any case, many institutions either have no security products or lack the ability or will to configure them properly. More importantly, if an attacker takes control of a computer system and wishes to cause maximum harm, his or her task is considerably more complex than causing the system to crash. To maximize harm in an ITS control system, for example, an attacker might attempt to alter the vehicle headway control software to cause simultaneous vehicle collisions system-wide. (Independent on-vehicle systems might preclude such an attack.)

Of course, carrying out such an attack would require substantial knowledge of the system's design and operation. Acquiring this knowledge is more difficult than breaking into a computer. It requires the support of an insider (in the ITS operation or the software vendor), access to maintenance documentation (probably stored on a computer that can be broken into), or substantial reverse engineering of software downloaded from the network under attack. An attack-development team would have to be as competent, patient, and detail oriented as any software product-development team.

The committee is not aware of any current plans for surface transportation systems that would be vulnerable to such attacks. Even the air traffic control system, which is far more highly automated and centralized than any part of the surface transportation infrastructure, is still relatively decentralized and retains the option for individual controllers to control traffic, albeit at reduced capacity. ITS technology may offer comparable levels of automated control in the future, but it seems likely that the highway infrastructure as a whole will remain distributed and decentralized and retain reduced-capacity fallback modes for the foreseeable future. Nevertheless, as infrastructure operators deploy higher levels of infrastructure-wide automation, they would be well advised to consider the need for the infrastructure to operate even if the control systems are degraded or unavailable.

In addition, wherever possible, operators should isolate control systems from public networks, such as the Internet or the public switched telephone network. Current trends in telecommunications make it very difficult to achieve complete isolation—for example, two otherwise separate circuits may happen to travel on the same fiber, or at least traverse the same bridge over a river—but intentional and unintentional connectivity should be minimized. As explained below, sharing a communications link (e.g., a fiber or a wireless connection) is less of a security concern than sharing a switching node in the network. If network access is provided, it should be limited, and the systems that provide access should be reviewed for options that provide unauthorized access.

In the long term, as control systems become more automated, the security consequences will vary depending on the type of technology used and on whether the automated control is centralized or distributed. One-of-a-kind software or hardware is often extremely expensive. Commercial, off-the-shelf (COTS) technology is cheaper, but commercial developers usually emphasize new features and rapid time-to-market rather than reliability or security. Centralized automation increases vulnerability to natural disasters, operator failures, and software bugs. Decentralized automation requires orchestrated cooperation among mutually suspicious systems, a task for which today's science and technology base is limited.

The security of information systems is discussed in much greater detail in a recent National Research Council report, *Trust in Cyberspace* (NRC, 1998).

Learning about Interdependencies from Accidents and Natural Disasters

In addition to the redundancy study suggested above, internal interdependencies of the surface transportation system can be identified and understood by analogy with lessons learned from accidents and natural disasters.

Most disasters, whether natural or caused by accidental or intentional human action, have been extensively studied after the fact. The committee is not aware, however, of any unified assessment of best practices and lessons learned, based on a large sample of disasters. (A recent study conducted at San Jose State University attempts such an assessment of four terrorist incidents [Mineta Institute, 1997].) A compendium of such postmortem analyses would be useful. It should focus on how surface transportation was affected and include an evaluation of successful and unsuccessful approaches to preventing or mitigating adverse consequences. It might be similar in some ways, though more general in scope, to information gathered by the National Bomb Data Center of the Federal Bureau of Investigation.

One incident that could be included is the multiple disaster on January 13, 1982, in Washington, D.C. Shortly after 4 o'clock on a Wednesday afternoon, an airplane crashed into the 14th Street Bridge, which carries the I-395 and US-1 highways. As a result, all 12 lanes of the busiest bridge across the Potomac were closed for several days. Just 30 minutes later, a train derailment blocked two of the city's three subway lines in both directions, again for several days. And at the same time, a major snowstorm affected road and highway traffic, as well as rescue and repair efforts. Another obvious candidate for analysis is the simultaneous damage to multiple highways often caused by major earthquakes (see Box 2-3).

"Y2K" computer problems associated with the year 2000, which have the advantage of occurring on a date that is known in advance, may provide interesting lessons about interdependencies in the cyber domain. These lessons could emerge from the many modeling and planning exercises that are being conducted before the event, as well as from the actual consequences. The analogy between Y2K and the threat of cyber attacks may be similar to the analogy between hazardous materials and the threat of chemical attacks.

Interdependencies with Other Infrastructure Sectors

The surface transportation system relies on a variety of other infrastructure sectors. The power grid, for example, is needed to run subway trains, traffic management systems, the cranes that load cargo vessels, the pumps that supply vehicles with gasoline and other fuels, and many other aspects of the system. All

BOX 2-3
The Impact of Earthquakes on Surface Transportation

The Northridge earthquake in 1994, which was centered 20 miles northwest of downtown Los Angeles, caused structural damage that cost an estimated $25 billion (Gordon et al., 1998). Four major highways were blocked, including sections of the Santa Monica Freeway (I-10, "the world's busiest freeway") and the Golden State Freeway (I-5, California's main north-south artery). Despite this damage, the surface transportation system showed remarkable resiliency. Freeway traffic was rerouted onto parallel local arteries. Many commuters adjusted their destinations and times of departure or found ways to telecommute. The use of commuter rail increased.

Similarly, the Loma Prieta earthquake in 1989 caused extensive damage to several highways, including the collapse of a section of the Bay Bridge, the major surface link between the northern San Francisco Peninsula and the rest of the country. To compensate, travelers made increased use of ferry service and the Bay Area Rapid Transit system, several major employers instituted shuttle services, and many commuters adjusted their routes and travel schedules.

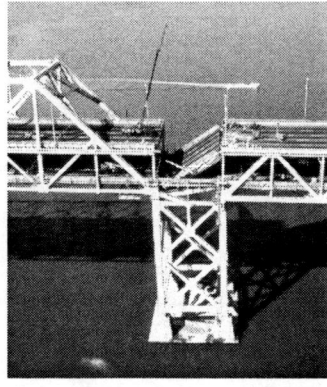

The collapsed section of the Bay Bridge after the 1989 Loma Prieta earthquake. Photo courtesy of E.V. Leyendecker, U.S. Geological Survey.

Natural disasters like these suggest that "transportation system redundancy and the ability of individuals to make a variety of short-term adjustments in travel patterns make rapid recovery possible even from major disasters" (Giuliano and Golob, 1998). There is good reason for optimism that the same would be true in the aftermath of a disaster caused by intentional hostile acts, such as bombings of highways or bridges. Intentional attacks and natural disasters may affect public confidence quite differently, however. After the December 1996 bombing of a Paris commuter train, for example, in which four were killed and 86 injured, restoration of normal service took only three days, but ridership did not return to its previous level for several months (U.S. Department of State, 1997; Aymeric, 1999).

Further analysis of past natural disasters and major accidents could be very helpful in understanding possible future hostile attacks, to identify both what can be done in advance to minimize vulnerability and what can be done after an incident occurs to mitigate the consequences. Despite a number of studies of individual disasters and an extensive literature on travel behavior under everyday conditions, "prior research on travel behavior responses to major disasters is virtually nonexistent" (Giuliano and Golob, 1998). Moreover, changing commuting patterns and the growing prevalence of telecommuting and online shopping may have important effects on travel behavior.

modes of transportation are becoming increasingly reliant on the information infrastructure, such as networked telecommunications, computer databases, and GPS. Attacks on these systems could have large-scale consequences for transportation, perhaps greater than the consequences of most direct attacks on transportation assets.

For example, a variety of communications technologies are important for surface transportation. Among these are GPS, used for navigation; satellite-based tracking systems used by some trucking companies; wired and wireless systems for command, control, and dispatch; communications links between video surveillance cameras and monitors; and voice communications between control centers and vehicle operators.

These systems can be attacked in two main ways: disrupting the link itself (e.g., severing a cable or jamming a radio signal) or disrupting the computer-controlled network nodes that perform signaling, routing, and database functions. Attacking the control nodes is potentially more damaging. For example, some taxi companies use a commercial wireless data service for dispatching. This service could be disrupted by jamming one or more base stations. But it would be much more effective to introduce or exploit a software bug in the mobile switching office to disrupt signaling protocols to base stations across a wide area.

Attacks on the communications services used by surface transportation could have serious consequences, but the committee agrees with the judgment of the DOT vulnerability assessment that the consequences would probably be inconveniences and economic losses rather than loss of life. The communications infrastructure itself is quite resilient, with redundant communications links and fallback navigational systems. Moreover, communications security concerns are not unique to the transportation sector. Communications service providers and equipment manufacturers are already actively seeking ways to protect their customers. DOT should keep informed of developments in this area (see Box 2-4), but its main role should be to learn from others and, where appropriate, transfer that knowledge to surface transportation owners and operators.

The situation is similar for most other infrastructure sectors with which transportation is interdependent. In general, DOT should remain aware of developments, learn from others, and transfer knowledge to surface transportation owners and operators, but not participate directly in R&D. However, the two studies suggested above—an assessment of strategic vulnerabilities and a compendium of lessons learned from past incidents—should certainly take into account interdependencies with other sectors. For example, it might be instructive to examine the impact on surface transportation of major power blackouts, such as the one in San Francisco in December 1998 that halted the Bay Area Rapid Transit subway system and many city buses and disabled traffic signals.

> **BOX 2-4**
> **Implications for Surface Transportation of**
> **Trends in Communications**
>
> Current developments in communications are primarily aimed at providing the following improvements:
>
> 1. higher data rates at lower cost
> 2. integrated services, such as voice, data, and video, over the same communications substrate, such as the Internet or other facilities managed by local operators
> 3. services to mobile and portable hosts
>
> The data rates required for control signaling are typically quite low, except perhaps for video monitoring, so Trend 1 is largely irrelevant for surface transportation. Trend 2 is relevant in that it may make purchasing data services from a communications service provider more attractive than building a private network. Trend 3 implies the possibility of using commercial wireless services, such as cellular or wireless local area networks, to transmit control information.

Special Circumstances

Another circumstance in which the impact of a point attack on surface transportation might be significantly magnified is if the target were critical to a nationally important function. A prime example of this would be an attack during a military emergency or during military preparations to respond to a potential emergency. An attack against the surface transportation system of a major port city responsible for moving military cargo, for example, could delay significantly the rapid response on which today's defense strategies depend.

Military logistics today depend heavily on commercial rail, truck, and port terminals.[3] Despite the resiliency of the transportation system, point attacks on major bridges or tunnels or fuel terminals could disrupt traffic for hours, perhaps even days. In the context of a military emergency or another crisis, a disruption that might be less significant under ordinary circumstances could have major consequences. An assessment of strategic vulnerabilities, by identifying key transportation nodes that lack redundant alternatives, would help to highlight potential situations of this kind.

---

[3] The military also relies on commercial air transport, but that is outside the scope of this report.

SUMMARY

Overall, the DOT vulnerability assessment is excellent, but it should not be a one-time effort. Attention to the following points will help improve future assessments:

- The basic assumptions and predicted consequences of each scenario should be given a further reality check, in cooperation with appropriate industry representatives.
- Further assessment of threat likelihood is highly desirable, although very difficult.
- A more complete, balanced, and clearly defined analysis of possible means of attack will be needed for future assessment efforts.
- Cyber and other attacks on the C^3 systems of surface transportation are given insufficient attention in the assessment. The discussion that does appear is focused too narrowly on the introduction of computer viruses.
- Chemical and biological vulnerabilities must be considered carefully and seriously—not left to others to worry about. Future assessment efforts should distinguish carefully between chemical attacks and biological attacks and between attacks involving agents with different properties.
- Strategic, systemic vulnerabilities deserve close attention. These may result from interdependencies within the surface transportation system, interdependencies with other infrastructure sectors, or special circumstances involving nationally important functions. To improve its understanding of these issues, DOT should undertake (1) a strategic assessment of the surface transportation system's redundancies and interdependencies, and (2) an analysis of lessons learned about impact and mitigation from past accidents and natural disasters.

3

Establishing a Research and Development Strategy

At this early stage in the establishment of an R&D program for surface transportation security, building a solid strategic basis for the program, including a clearly thought out process for conducting it, is more important than identifying a detailed agenda of R&D topics. It may be tempting, given the importance of the problem, to rush into efforts to find near-term solutions. Nevertheless, because the security of the surface transportation infrastructure is a continuing, long-term concern, and the appropriate R&D responses to it are not yet well defined, a general strategy should be established and clarified first.

The surface transportation system and its security needs are so wide ranging and diverse that creating and maintaining a balanced, systematic R&D strategy will be a continuing challenge. The approach taken should be dynamic and able to evolve over time as the situation changes. Its perspective should encompass the surface transportation system as a whole, not transportation modes individually. The strategy should include both near-term and long-term efforts and should address both point vulnerabilities and system-wide strategic vulnerabilities.

This chapter presents the study's recommendations for such a strategy. Rather than choosing among the many promising R&D topics, it describes a process for making those choices—how to define DOT's role, how to maintain a balanced and systematic program, how to set priorities, how to make sure that the technologies and processes developed are appropriate for the intended users.

The recommended approach, a standard methodology used in systems engineering,[1] consists of five fundamental steps:

1. *Defining* the problem, the objectives, and the criteria for evaluating success or failure
2. *Identifying* ways to meet the objectives, namely potential R&D projects
3. *Evaluating* the alternatives identified in Step 2 against the objectives defined in Step 1
4. *Deciding* on a course of action
5. *Implementing* the decision

DOT itself is best placed to decide how to organize these steps internally, assign responsibilities for managing the various elements, and ensure their coordination with other agencies and with owners and operators throughout the transportation sector. As noted elsewhere in this report, no matter what approach is adopted, the crosscutting problem of improving security should not be divided up according to transportation modes. Rather, part of DOT's strategy should be to assign lead responsibility for security R&D to a single person or office. Other changes in organization or approach may also be necessary to implement certain elements of the strategy, such as the involvement of owners and operators. Beyond these recommendations, however, it would be outside this study's charge to take a position on organizational or procedural matters that are internal to DOT.

DEFINING THE PROBLEM AND OBJECTIVES

The first step, defining the problem and objectives, is critical for everything that follows because it determines the criteria for evaluating potential R&D projects and making decisions. Because this is also the most difficult step, it should be given high priority and undertaken with great care. A common error is to pay insufficient attention to this step, or even ignore it completely, and jump directly to the identification of possible solutions. Perhaps thinking up potential solutions gives one a sense that rapid progress is being made and appears to provide more scope for creativity, but making that error can have serious consequences. That is why the main focus of this study is on developing a strategy for R&D rather than providing a specific agenda of R&D projects.

Defining the problem begins with identifying the needs that generated it, such as the need to prevent attacks or mitigate their impact, and describing the circumstances in which the problem exists. (The categorization of security needs will be used later to categorize R&D responses. See Box 3-1.) In general terms,

---

[1] The field of systems engineering has developed an extensive body of literature and experience over the past 50 years or so. For readers unfamiliar with the field, Appendix A briefly summarizes some key points and provides references for further reading.

> **BOX 3-1**
> **A Matrix for Categorizing R&D Topics in Surface Transportation Security**
>
> | | Type of Attack | | | | |
> |---|---|---|---|---|---|
> | Response Area | Biological | Chemical | Cyber/C^3 | Explosive | General |
> | Prevention | . | . | . | . | . |
> | Mitigation | . | . | . | . | . |
> | Monitoring | . | . | . | . | . |
> | Recovery | . | . | . | . | . |
> | Investigation | . | . | . | . | . |
> | Systems Responses | . | . | . | . | . |
>
> This matrix is a framework for identifying and evaluating possible R&D topics. The columns represent the major types of attack and the rows the major categories of R&D response to improve security against those attacks. Note that transportation modes are intentionally not separated from each other. The following definitions of the response categories are explained further, with examples, in Chapter 4:
>
> *Prevention:* preventing an attacker from carrying out an attack.
> *Mitigation:* reducing the harmful impact of an attack as it occurs and in its immediate aftermath.
> *Monitoring:* recognizing that an attack is taking place, identifying its type and magnitude, and predicting and monitoring its development.
> *Recovery:* returning to normal operation after an attack is over.
> *Investigation:* identifying what happened in an attack, how it happened, and who was responsible.
> *Systems responses:* ensuring that elements of the system function together properly and learning more about the problem to improve overall system effectiveness.
>
> Crosscutting needs, such as education, training, and technology transfer, do not appear in the matrix as separate categories. They should be integral components of all responses in all categories.

the problem under consideration here is to construct a program of R&D that will improve the security of the surface transportation system. Describing this problem will require identifying technological and procedural security needs that are not currently being met. It will also require identifying a variety of other factors: the available funding, the nature of the threat, the relevant R&D already being conducted elsewhere, competing transportation goals such as openness and accessibility and efficiency, societal and legal constraints on approaches to security, and so on. Clear and accurate descriptions of these factors will provide useful limits on both the problem and its solution.

The nature of the threat is an important aspect of the problem. Planning and carrying out an attack are costly to an attacker, both financially and in the risk of discovery. The size, complexity, and expense of each potential attack correspond to the attacker's risk and the resources required. One cannot necessarily predict an attacker's sensitivity to cost and risk or his level of motivation and resolve, but nevertheless, potential security countermeasures should be characterized according the level of attack they address and the level of risk that would remain after they have been deployed.

The analysis should then proceed to establish objectives that will later serve as criteria for evaluating potential solutions. It may be helpful to picture these objectives as a hierarchical tree, with an overall system goal at the root of the tree, midlevel objectives branching out from it, and quantifiable measures of performance as the leaves.

A key element should be a clear definition of what DOT seeks to accomplish by its R&D activities in surface transportation security. DOT's answer to this question should include the following system-level goals:

- a comprehensive understanding of the surface transportation system's point and systemic vulnerabilities to hostile attack
- a comprehensive understanding of existing security technologies and processes and how to apply them effectively to surface transportation
- the development of new security technologies and processes in response to specific, clearly identified vulnerabilities that are unique to surface transportation
- the implementation of effective security technologies and processes by surface transportation owners and operators in such a way that vulnerabilities to attack are reduced without significantly compromising other transportation goals

Note that these objectives are likely to lead to a diverse program that includes many types of R&D: hardware, software, and system development; technology evaluation and testing; pilot programs; paper studies; and technology transfer.

Implementing the R&D results will present many challenges, including cost, potential delays to passengers or cargo, privacy concerns, the balance of perceived benefits and perceived risks, and the balance between protecting against attacks and disrupting ongoing activities. Some of these factors, particularly cost and effectiveness, may be difficult to determine in advance—that is the nature of R&D—but objectives for them should nevertheless be considered as carefully as possible. For example, most people will never experience an actual incident, so it is highly desirable to build security measures into everyday operations as "just a good way of doing business." Moreover, some security measures can have positive side effects on everyday operations, such as reducing thefts of cargo or losses of passenger baggage. The value of such dual-use benefits—which serve a business purpose, as well as promoting security, and thus turn security from a cost to an asset—should be recognized explicitly in setting objectives.

Defining the Department of Transportation's Role

An important factor in defining the objectives is a clear understanding of DOT's proper role. The federal government already conducts extensive R&D on counterterrorism and related aspects of infrastructure protection. This work is spread among a variety of agencies. The R&D resources of some of these agencies, such as the Departments of Defense and Energy, are much greater than those that DOT is likely to devote to security R&D for surface transportation. Nevertheless, DOT has an important role to play. Clearly identifying that role, a niche that capitalizes on other agencies' efforts without reinventing the wheel, will be critical to the effectiveness of DOT's program of R&D for surface transportation security. For each potential R&D project the question must be, Is DOT the right agency to address this particular aspect of the problem?

Even in some important areas, where surface transportation is clearly vulnerable, the answer to this question will be No. For example, many elements of the surface transportation system are becoming increasingly automated and reliant on computers and communications for their continuing operation. As this trend continues and even accelerates, the transportation infrastructure will become increasingly vulnerable to a cyber attack on the telecommunications system. For example, many traffic operations centers in urban areas transmit control information and traffic data over ordinary telephone lines, so the security of the telephone network is certainly an important concern for surface transportation. But its importance is by no means unique to surface transportation, and so it would make little sense for DOT to take on this challenge. Similarly, hardening the structure of railway or bus stations against bomb blasts is probably not very different from hardening the structure of other public buildings, so general R&D on structural hardening may be best left to others. The objectives that DOT establishes, against which potential R&D projects in surface transportation security will be evaluated, must be able to identify such situations, which will not always be as clear cut as these examples.

DOT does have a vital role to play. Within DOT, since the early 1970s the Federal Aviation Administration has conducted a significant and valuable program on weapon and explosives detection and other techniques to protect air transportation. Moreover, DOT has a long history of responding effectively to natural disasters, which are in many ways a similar problem to intentional attacks, though the emphasis of the response may be different. (For example, mitigation and rapid recovery are important in both cases, but security measures may also include prevention and forensic investigation.) DOT has a similarly valuable R&D role in protecting surface transportation against hostile attacks.

One likely niche for DOT is evaluating transportation applications of technology developed elsewhere and helping to transfer promising technology to the transportation sector. For example, the Department of Defense, the Department of Energy, and others have already developed a number of systems for detecting chemical agents, but many challenging problems arise when these systems are used in enclosed spaces, such as subways. The rate of false alarms must be much lower in a subway than in many other places, even other large civilian facilities such as office buildings, because in those facilities alarms and evacuations cause only localized disruption. In contrast, even if only one subway station is affected directly, operations are likely to be disrupted system-wide. At the same time, the confined air in an urban subway is likely to be a very difficult background against which to identify hazardous chemicals. Thus perhaps DOT has an important role to play in evaluating the available products for subway use—are their false-alarm rates acceptably low despite the heavy chemical and biological background contained in ordinary subway air? This is just one example of the useful role DOT could play in collecting and disseminating guidelines on security best practices for surface transportation operators.

DOT's role will also be influenced by the fact that some special characteristics of surface transportation systems may not be adequately addressed elsewhere. In the case of subways, for example, the piston action of trains as they pass through tunnels could provide attackers with a uniquely effective means of dispersing a chemical or biological agent throughout a city. DOT might therefore consider a variety of subway-specific R&D responses, such as developing airflow barriers, modeling aerosol dispersion in tunnels and ventilation systems (which is already being done at DOT and elsewhere), or measuring the baseline levels of chemical species and microbes already present in ordinary subway air. In the case of railway and bus stations, even though they may present no transportation-unique security issues in structural design, the potential for a bombing to disrupt the rest of the transportation system may suggest some important R&D topics for systems modeling. Or if there are aspects of R&D on bomb-protecting structures that focus specifically on bridges and tunnels, two elements that are essentially unique to transportation, it might make sense for DOT to focus R&D in those areas.

Setting Priorities

A final vital aspect of setting objectives is the establishment of criteria for prioritizing R&D outcomes. A huge variety of security R&D projects can be imagined that would all be desirable and appropriate for DOT if infinite resources were available. How should DOT select from such a list? There are many possible criteria.

One obvious approach is to give the most likely threats the highest priority. This would require an assessment of risk, beyond the assessment of vulnerability discussed in Chapter 2. For example, domestic "patriot" or "militia" groups have specifically advocated attacks against the rail infrastructure. If that threat is considered credible and serious, perhaps an emphasis on protecting rail transport might be appropriate. But this approach is not enough. In many cases, if not most cases, reliable threat information is simply not available. Even the best intelligence efforts have trouble identifying threats from lone individuals, and in any case, the greatest threat is likely to be unanticipated.

Moreover, a security R&D program must look toward future needs. Threats change much more quickly than vulnerabilities. Because R&D results take time to produce and implement, DOT's program must provide for the likelihood that today's threat will not be the same as tomorrow's. This suggests a bias toward solutions with broad applicability. Yes, it is essential to continue the ongoing efforts by various agencies to develop better threat information, and any threat information that is available would certainly be an important input to the process of R&D prioritization, but other approaches are also needed.

The objectives of an R&D strategy should include factors based on the answers to such questions as these:

- If a threat does materialize, how serious is its potential impact on people, property, and society? Would the consequences be so disastrous that we must not ignore the threat even if it appears highly unlikely?
- Where can additional R&D resources result in the most improvement per dollar? Is the rate of progress in this area limited by the state of technology or the availability of funding?
- Is this an area where a modest R&D investment could make a significant advance toward solving a problem completely?
- Would R&D in this area have other benefits (such as improving security against theft or robbery, or preventing accidents) even if the threat of a hostile attack never materialized? Dual-use results might have a significantly greater chance of being accepted and implemented by transportation owners and operators.
- Would R&D in this area respond to just one type of vulnerability, or many?
- What related R&D topics are other agencies investigating that DOT could use to increase the return on its own (probably modest) R&D resources?
- What R&D topics are other agencies *not* investigating, and do they include transportation-specific needs that will be ignored if DOT does nothing?
- Are there useful technologies, already developed by other agencies, that require integration before being transferred to the transportation sector?

Based on the answers to the first question, DOT might choose to prioritize R&D opportunities by the magnitude of the vulnerability they would address. Or based on answers to the second and third questions, DOT might choose to prioritize R&D projects according to inherent "ripeness for progress," perhaps as determined by peer review in the R&D community. Choices such as these are part of the process of defining the problem and setting objectives.

IDENTIFYING POTENTIAL ALTERNATIVES

The second step of the recommended strategy is to examine as wide a range of potential solutions as possible. This study has intentionally avoided dividing its subject matter up according to the various modes of transportation. The process DOT chooses for identifying potential R&D projects should do the same. Although most transportation-related R&D is organized and funded according to transportation mode, there is so much synergy and overlap among the security concerns of the different modes that such a division in this case would be artificial and deleterious.

Instead, DOT should categorize potential R&D topics according to a matrix like the one shown in Box 3-1, with each element of the matrix representing a combination of a particular type of attack (without regard to the type of target) and a particular type of response. This approach has several attractions, both for considering processes and strategies and for considering individual R&D projects. First, it ensures completeness; because each column describes a threat and each row a response, one can quickly evaluate the coverage of threats with research in each response area. Second, it provides a flexible way to define both programs (strategic plans) and projects (tactical plans). Third, it can be used to assess quickly the technological status of existing responses to various threats. Fourth, it provides a convenient communications vehicle because of its simple two-dimensional structure. Finally, it is both stable and robust; the row and column categories will remain relevant for defining research strategies and tactics for the foreseeable future, and when changes do occur they can be easily accommodated by adding rows or columns, with no need to reorganize what was there before.

Each proposed alternative must be described in sufficient detail that it can be evaluated against the objectives. Essentially this means that, for each potential R&D project, all relevant consequences should be described concretely—not only security consequences, but also more general consequences, such as the cost and practicality of implementation, the effect on travel time and convenience, potential legal or privacy concerns, and so on. At a minimum, potential projects should be described in sufficient detail that they can be understood clearly by whoever would ultimately have to implement them. (Too much detail, of course, could delay the whole exercise and increase its cost and complexity. Striking an appropriate balance, however, should not be too difficult.)

EVALUATING ALTERNATIVES

In the evaluation step of the strategy, each alternative should be formally measured against the objectives defined at the beginning of the process. That is, once DOT has systematically identified a wide variety of potential R&D projects, it must assess the impact each would have if it were successful and its results were implemented. Here again, impact means not only the impact on security, but also the broader impact on the transportation system and society as a whole. For example, the evaluation in this step should include trade-offs such as the balance of security against cost and inconvenience. A sensitivity analysis should be included to identify how changes in assumptions would change the evaluation.

Establishing the capability to conduct such an evaluation is not a simple task. For example, one of the criteria developed during the problem definition phase is sure to be the specificity of the project to DOT's unique role and responsibilities. Evaluating projects against this criterion will clearly require effective coordination and information sharing between DOT and other federal and state agencies. Because of the wide range of work being done and the variety of agencies involved, this will be a significant challenge. The Critical Infrastructure Coordinating Group's interagency working group on R&D is one important mechanism for coordination, and DOT should continue to place a high priority on its participation in that group. In addition, the coordinating role of the Technical Support Working Group should be very useful, although that organization is not involved in all projects. The committee understands that the Federal Aviation Administration and the DOT Office of Intelligence and Security participate regularly in Technical Support Working Group subgroups. That participation should continue, and if possible, other DOT agencies involved in security R&D for surface transportation should also participate.

There are a variety of ways DOT can improve its capability to evaluate the priority-setting criteria discussed above. For example, it might choose to intensify its efforts to develop threat intelligence. Or (as suggested in Chapter 2) it might conduct more analysis of past incidents of various types to assess the effectiveness of various alternatives. Or it might convene workshops to elicit expert technical input on the probable success or effectiveness of various R&D approaches. (These workshops could also be a good way to involve owners and operators.)

Some form of modeling or simulation is often used in evaluating complex situations. Evaluation has received more attention in the systems engineering literature than any other step of the recommended strategy, and that attention has generated considerable controversy because sophisticated techniques have often been applied to problems with poorly specified or inconsistent objectives. Sophisticated evaluation techniques do not guarantee good results unless the basic description of the problem is clear, consistent, and complete.

DECIDING ON A COURSE OF ACTION

The fourth step, deciding on a course of action, means more than just selecting a portfolio of R&D projects. For example, a potential project might be evaluated as important and likely to succeed but not appropriate for DOT. In that case, the right course of action would involve coordinating with other agencies to make sure they are addressing the problem and are aware of its transportation-specific aspects. DOT must be able to tell other agencies that "this needs to be done, but we aren't the ones to do it." DOT's overall R&D strategy for surface transportation security should include planning for this situation as well as planning for DOT itself to conduct R&D.

Decision making has received considerable attention in the systems-engineering literature. Although the evaluation process involves rating each alternative against each objective, these ratings usually do not produce a unique solution. Usually multiple objectives compete with each other, and no single alternative is dominant on every scale. A decision model is therefore necessary to rank the alternatives. Theoretically, the soundest approach is based on utility functions (Keeney and Raiffa, 1976), but this approach is too expensive and time-consuming for most organizations. The simplest alternative is to provide managers with graphical displays of the ratings of each alternative against each objective and allow them to make the final selection. Other approaches assign a simple weight to each objective and provide a single overall score for each alternative. Clearly DOT's choice of a decision model should depend on the resources available and the importance attached to each decision.

IMPLEMENTING THE PLAN

The final step is implementation, which may involve communicating decisions at various levels inside and outside the government, developing budgets and schedules, obtaining resources, and assigning responsibilities. Note that for surface transportation security, implementation means much more than instituting the R&D program. The real goal, of course, is to ensure that security solutions are implemented in the surface transportation system, not just to develop technologies and processes for their own sake. Thus implementing the R&D plan will have to include ensuring the implementation of R&D results.

Accomplishing that goal will require commitment by high-level management, incorporation of R&D results into ongoing agency programs, and user acceptance of the technologies and processes developed. It will also depend on raising the transportation community's awareness of how new approaches and techniques can improve security. Buy-in within DOT, both by top-level officials and by program managers throughout the department, will be essential for R&D investments to be made wisely and their results widely disseminated. Buy-in by state and local transportation agencies will be equally important. Finally, and perhaps most important, success will depend on ensuring that transportation system owners and operators endorse and help shape DOT's R&D program.

Involving Owners and Operators

Involving owners and operators in the R&D process is essential to achieving their acceptance of its results and is therefore critical to the success of the strategy's implementation step. DOT should place considerable emphasis on this involvement. Owners and operators can provide a critical, real-world perspective on the balance of costs and benefits, on issues involving human factors, on the dynamics of the industry, on how these factors may influence a technology's acceptance, and on how new technologies can be managed successfully in the context of the existing infrastructure. All these considerations are important elements in defining R&D priorities and determining a concept's potential for successful implementation.

One mechanism for involving owners and operators is to hold regular workshops, review panels, and other meetings. A model for this approach could be the workshop on chemical and biological threats to transportation held in September 1998 at the DOT Volpe Center in Cambridge, Massachusetts, and the planned follow-on symposium with broader participation. Similar activities could be undertaken in other technical areas, such as cyber security or protection against bomb blasts. Another model could be the Gordon Research Conference on Illicit Substance Detection, held in August 1998, which also focused on chemical and biological attacks. A valuable feature of that meeting was the opportunity it provided for leading researchers to come together with those whose main concerns are policy making and implementation. Interactions like these build a strong foundation for future information sharing and improve researchers' understanding of government and industry needs. Strong industrial participation is particularly important for outcomes to be in owners' and operators' best interests, as well as the national interest. Strong participation by state departments of transportation would help convince owners and operators of the seriousness of the issues and thus encourage implementation.

Technology transfer should be a consideration from the very beginning of each project. Potential technology users should be involved in all phases of the program, from the planning and development of fundamental strategy to the selection and continuing oversight of individual projects. This bottom-up approach will help ensure that the projects selected reflect a realistic view of the operational situation in the real world of surface transportation. For example, in a major ferry operation the turnaround time is often very rapid, with hundreds of vehicles and people being unloaded and loaded in a period of perhaps 15 minutes. A vehicle or baggage scanning system designed to detect explosives would be impractical for such an application if it introduced even a small delay in the time required to board each vehicle or passenger. Involving someone with direct experience of ferry operations would help to identify such problems early in the process. Similarly, transit systems and parking facilities have ticket turnstiles and control gates that single out individual travelers or vehicles. Perhaps chemical sensing systems could be incorporated into this equipment to alert security personnel, but unless operators were involved in the development process, it would be easy to develop a product that no one would use. (Would maintenance be practical? Would the system cause delays for travelers? What should the response be in the event of an alarm, and would the false-alarm rate be acceptably low?) Examples can easily be imagined for each mode of transportation and each type of potential R&D response.

DOT should undertake an aggressive, ongoing campaign to educate transportation owners and operators about threats, vulnerabilities, and R&D results. The outreach effort could be generic, or separate teams could be assembled to specialize in the concerns of urban transit, say, or pipelines or railroads. Incidents particularly relevant to the target audience (such as the sarin attack in the Tokyo subway, for a transit audience) could be used to motivate operators to participate. Feedback from the campaign would help DOT identify technological and procedural security needs and useful areas for further R&D, as well as how operator perceptions and attitudes are likely to affect implementation. This would help DOT keep its R&D strategy dynamic and responsive in the long term. Moreover, the resulting heightened awareness of security issues could encourage operators to increase their security efforts using existing techniques, even before any R&D came to fruition.

Active outreach would have several side benefits. First, by creating a group of interested stakeholders out in the field, it would establish a pool of likely early adopters or beta-testers of new systems resulting from R&D. Second, by building relationships with owners and operators, it would facilitate the provision of other security-related support, such as new equipment or training. Last but not least, by building wider awareness and support, it could strengthen DOT's argument for increasing the resources allocated to security R&D.

DOT should also consider outreach and education directed toward users of transportation services. Ultimately, travelers and shippers will be the ones who decide whether to pay higher prices so that owners and operators can recover the cost of added security measures. Outreach to users would have to be designed carefully to avoid either undermining public confidence in the safety and security of the current surface transportation system or desensitizing users to security concerns by "crying wolf" when actual incidents are admittedly infrequent.

Involving owners and operators in the R&D process may also build acceptance of the reality of the threat that the R&D results are designed to protect against. Many surface transportation operators believe that hostile attacks against their facilities are unlikely, and at least for most of them, this perception is probably correct. Persuading them that security should be a real concern and that security measures will be cost-effective for their facilities will be a challenge (see Box 3-2). Increased dissemination of intelligence information to major players in the surface transportation industry could increase their acceptance of the need for new technologies and processes, but direct involvement is key.

All these efforts to involve owners and operators must be taken seriously as a fundamental part of the R&D strategy. Stakeholders should be considered more than just a source of input and ideas. They should have a real say in which R&D projects are undertaken and how they are conducted. Only genuine, two-way communication will ensure that security concerns become an integral part of system design and day-to-day operations.

PROTECTING SENSITIVE INFORMATION

As DOT builds up its R&D in surface transportation security, it will encounter a growing need to protect information that is sensitive, but not classified. For example, increased dissemination of intelligence to transportation operators, as recommended above, may be problematic unless access to that intelligence can be controlled. This concern is not reflected directly in the recommended five-stage strategic process, but resolving it is vital so that the process can have full access to relevant information sources and result in effective implementation. Indeed, this issue arose several times just during the course of this study.

Existing guidelines for the release of information provide no mechanism for solving this problem. For example, DOT might wish to provide sensitive information to a variety of people with legitimate and constructive reasons to use it, such as individuals responsible for security in major transportation companies— or for that matter, the committee that prepared this report. Currently, however, unless the information is actually classified, there is no legal means to do this without also making it available to the public at large under the requirements of laws such as the Freedom of Information Act.

Some agencies have already resolved this dilemma. For example, the Federal Aviation Administration, which has been struggling with security issues for much longer than have DOT's surface transportation components, has recourse to a regulation known as 14 CFR 191, which protects information resulting from R&D on aviation security. Agency officials can disseminate "191" information to appropriate individuals within airlines, airports, security equipment manufacturers, local law enforcement and emergency services organizations, security policy analysts, and so on without rendering it subject to general public disclosure.

As DOT expands its R&D activities in surface transportation security, information protection is likely to become increasingly worrisome. DOT should consider urging the Congress to provide legal authority for a regulation similar to 14 CFR 191.

BOX 3-2
Operators' Perceptions of Threats

The committee visited several surface transportation facilities during the course of this study. A common characteristic of these sites was their low level of security against hostile attacks. This is generally the situation except at ports of entry, where the Immigration and Naturalization Service and the Customs Service have placed terrorism higher on their agenda. The infrastructure operators with whom the committee spoke during the site visits perceived a low level of threat. They were primarily concerned about theft or robbery of cash, personal property, and cargo. Where the committee did encounter airport-style security equipment—at the passenger embarkation point for a cruise ship—it was applied inconsistently. Passengers were made to walk through metal detectors and their hand luggage was x-rayed, but their checked luggage was not examined at all, even though it would be freely available to them once they were on board. The gap between today's level of security and even a modest level of protection against hostile attack appears to be wide indeed.

Based on this experience, it appears that operators' perceptions of threat are likely to have a major impact on the deployment of any products of the R&D described in this report. Governments may mandate security measures, but these requirements have historically followed incidents rather than anticipated them. In the absence of legislation, operators will deploy only the security measures they believe to be cost effective.

The importance of cost effectiveness for owners and operators cannot be overstated. This is not an abstract or hypothetical concern. For example, throughout the 1980s, sponsors of research on computer and network security funded and encouraged the development of technologies that were intended to be highly effective against hostile attacks on computers and networks. However, the funding agencies were unable to convince private-sector suppliers and users of computers and networks that the threat justified integration of these technologies into high-volume products or their application to commercial or government systems. As a result, the research funds expended had little direct impact on the security of real systems (NRC, 1998). DOT should not follow the same path by funding security solutions that are not supported by owners and operators and thus are never deployed.

One way to help ensure that R&D expenditures ultimately yield real security improvements is to support dual-use technologies that can address both hostile threats against infrastructure and other disruptions, such as robberies, accidents, or natural disasters. An example of this effect is the experience of commercial airlines, for which the expense and complication of security-driven requirements for baggage tracking and passenger identification have resulted in less luggage lost and fewer illegal transfers of nontransferable tickets.

SUMMARY

Building a solid strategic basis is the most important task at this early stage in DOT's establishment of an R&D program for surface transportation security. That strategy should be a systematic process consisting of five fundamental steps:

1. *Defining* the problem, the objectives, and the criteria for evaluating success or failure
2. *Identifying* ways to meet the objectives, namely potential R&D projects
3. *Evaluating* the alternatives identified in Step 2 against the objectives defined in Step 1
4. *Deciding* on a course of action
5. *Implementing* the decision

The implementation of this strategy should incorporate the following key features:

- Because improving security is a crosscutting problem, DOT should not break up its efforts in this area according to transportation modes.
- DOT should clearly identify and understand its role in security R&D and how that role meshes with work being done by other agencies.
- As a framework for identifying and evaluating potential R&D topics, DOT should categorize topics according to the type of attack to which they respond and the type of response to which they are directed: prevention, mitigation, monitoring, recovery, investigation, or systems.
- DOT should make strenuous efforts to increase the involvement of transportation owners and operators. Their serious involvement in all stages of the program will be critical to successful implementation.
- To meet the growing need to protect information that is sensitive, but not classified, DOT should consider urging the Congress to provide legal authority similar to the regulation 14 CFR 191, which protects information on aviation security.

4
Applying the Methodology: Some Specific Research and Development Topics

The focus of this report so far has been on establishing a firm strategic basis for R&D on surface transportation security. A fundamental conclusion of the study is that addressing broad issues of strategy should be DOT's first priority in responding to concerns in this area. This chapter presents some examples of specific R&D opportunities. The selection is not meant to be comprehensive, or even necessarily to represent the topics with the highest priority, but rather to illustrate the application of the methodology recommended in Chapter 3 and indicate where that approach might lead. Some topics are new R&D; others are technologies or processes that already exist in other contexts but have not been applied to improving the security of surface transportation.

The committee believes that the topics presented are promising, but DOT should conduct a full evaluation of its own using the framework of the careful, rigorous strategy that this report recommends. Inclusion in this chapter is not intended as a substitute for such evaluation. For example, more work is needed to determine how each potential project would fit into the broader picture of work being done at other agencies. Indeed, it would probably be unwise for DOT to initiate R&D on as many different topics as are presented here, even if it determined that they were all individually useful and appropriate. Table 4-1 illustrates how some of the topics discussed fit into the matrix structure that is part of the strategy.

Even though this chapter is only a preliminary application of the strategy and is intended primarily to illustrate the methodology, several of its themes are sure to reemerge when a more complete and thorough evaluation is conducted. They include the following, some of which have already been mentioned:

TABLE 4-1   Illustration of the Matrix Categorization of R&D Topics

	Type of Attack				
Response	Biological	Chemical	Cyber and C^3	Physical	General
Prevention	platform-edge doors	prerelease detection	software firewalls	explosives detection	study of redundancies
Mitigation	low-tech best practices	protective aerosols	ITS graceful degradation	construction design	lessons from natural disasters
Monitoring	—	chemical detector evaluation	identification of abnormal activity	—	video surveillance
Recovery	decontamination	decontamination	—	rapid bridge repairs	bandwidth reservation
Investigation	—	—	logging	—	best practices
Systems Integration	dispersion modeling	dispersion modeling	best practices	—	incident management

Note: This table categorizes some of the technologies and processes discussed in this chapter according to type of attack and type of R&D response. Also included, to show how they fit into the matrix concept, are two studies discussed in Chapter 2 (a compendium of lessons learned from past natural disasters and accidents and a study of redundancies and interdependencies). This is not a complete or exclusive list, just some examples arranged to illustrate the matrix approach.

- the value of taking a *dual-use* approach, in which security objectives are furthered at the same time as other transportation goals
- the potential for more use of *modeling* to develop a better understanding of the scope of the security problem
- the importance of DOT's role in developing and disseminating information about *best practices* that use existing technologies and processes, including low-technology alternatives
- the need to consider security as *part of a broader picture*, not a wholly new and different problem, but one that is similar and closely connected to the transportation community's previous experience in responding to concerns about safety, natural disasters, and hazardous materials

The strategy begins with definition of the problem and establishment of objectives. As discussed in Chapter 3, DOT's broad objectives for R&D efforts in surface transportation security should resemble the following:

- a comprehensive understanding of the surface transportation system's point and systemic vulnerabilities to hostile attack
- a comprehensive understanding of existing security technologies and processes and how to apply them effectively to surface transportation
- the development of new security technologies and processes in response to specific, clearly identified vulnerabilities that are unique to surface transportation
- the implementation of effective security technologies and processes by surface transportation owners and operators in such a way that vulnerabilities to attack are reduced without significantly compromising other transportation goals

The first of these objectives is closely related to the discussion in Chapter 2, and the two studies recommended there follow directly from it. The fourth objective should be an overarching theme of the entire R&D program and how it is implemented. The second and third objectives, which relate to R&D on specific technologies and processes, will be the main subject of this chapter. The focus will be primarily on applying the second and third steps of the strategy (i.e., the identification and evaluation of alternatives).

The six categories of R&D response (the rows of the matrix) can be used as midlevel objectives that are subordinate to the broad objectives listed above but are still fairly generic. That is, the vulnerabilities referred to in the broad objectives can be addressed in six ways that divide the problem into more manageable pieces. The remainder of this chapter is organized according to these six categories.

More topics are presented in some response categories than in others. This should not be taken to mean that those categories are more important. Indeed, response areas for which *few* suggestions appear may sometimes be the ones where the *most* work is needed to identify possible solutions.

PREVENTION

Technologies and processes in the "prevention" category should address the objective of preventing a potential attacker from carrying out a successful attack. (As discussed previously, they should also be evaluated against a host of other objectives, such as their cost, ease of implementation, effect on competing transportation goals, and so on. These other objectives apply in every category, and although this remark will not be repeated in each section of the chapter, it should not be forgotten.)

Examples include physical security—"guns, guards, and gates"—software to detect and prevent unauthorized computer access or the transmission of computer viruses, and sensing equipment to detect bombs or other threats before an incident occurs. Some options are generally applicable; others apply only to certain types of attack.

Generally Applicable Techniques

Fences and other physical barriers could keep potential attackers (of all types) away from vulnerable locations. There may be R&D opportunities in facility design to enhance the effectiveness of such barriers. Those opportunities would only be appropriate for DOT to the extent that the design issues are unique to transportation facilities, but DOT could play a role in disseminating design best practices to the transportation community.

Another option could be video monitoring, perhaps employing "smart" video, to help identify an imminent attack before it takes place. Smart video monitors might be able to automatically identify shapes or motions that are associated with suspicious objects or activities. This capability is currently quite limited but should improve with advances in image recognition and video processing. The Defense Advanced Research Projects Agency sponsors R&D in this area, and although video monitoring is far from unique to DOT's niche, DOT could seek to involve the transportation community. For example, a research group could use a transportation application to test its experimental algorithms.

Biological and Chemical Attacks

One approach to the prevention of biological or chemical attacks could be controlling or monitoring potential agents or their manufacturing precursors. For example, R&D could evaluate the feasibility of establishing and maintaining a database of the purchasers of certain chemicals. Possession of certain microorganisms and biotoxins already requires registration with the Centers for Disease Control and Prevention, and their transfer requires that both shipper and receiver file forms (IOM and NRC, 1999). There seems to be little here that is unique to DOT, however.

Another approach to preventing biological and chemical attacks would be to detect the presence of threatening substances before an attack actually released them. R&D in this area might be similar to the Federal Aviation Administration's work on detecting chemical traces of explosives on the outside of baggage to prevent explosive devices from being loaded onto aircraft. Detecting unintended traces of biological or chemical agents may be more difficult than detecting explosives, however. Unless these agents are kept contained with extreme care, any potential attacker will probably be killed by them before he or she can launch an attack. Measures of performance of detection systems could include speed and convenience of operation, ease of maintenance, and the rates of detection and false alarm for various levels of simulated threat. This type of detection is probably a long-term research problem, however, and work at this stage is likely to be broadly applicable in a variety of settings. If that is correct, seeking a transportation-specific niche could be premature. Rather than trying to develop this technology on its own, a more appropriate eventual role for DOT is likely to be evaluating the suitability of technologies developed elsewhere for use in specific surface transportation contexts.

Cyber and C^3 Attacks

R&D topics that could result in improved techniques for resisting cyber and C^3 attacks include improved software firewall technologies, hardware and software architectures and associated system designs that could confine the impact of malicious or flawed programs, improved integration of high-performance encryption into networks and systems, and improved security and configuration management tools for distributed computer systems. Most of these topics are already being addressed by research at federal agencies. Measures of performance for them are admittedly difficult to construct (except for the usual factors, such as cost, ease of implementation, and impact on other transportation goals). One possible measure could be the rate of successful attack in a red-team exercise.

Physical Attacks

The Federal Aviation Administration has a long-standing R&D program on explosives and weapons detection. DOT may find R&D opportunities in adapting that type of technology, which is currently directed toward prevention of airplane bombings and hijackings, for use in surface transportation settings. Adaptation would be an extremely difficult challenge, however, for most parts of the surface transportation system, because traveler access is generally much less controlled than in aviation. There are some exceptions, such as when the objective is to detect large threat quantities. For example, at least two companies have developed drive-through inspection systems for fully loaded trucks and cargo containers that can scan for explosives at a rate of 25 to 30 trucks per hour—too slow for general use on highways, but perhaps acceptable at selected locations, such as border crossings.

In some surface transportation situations, dogs are already commonly used for drug detection. For example, dogs are used at some freight ports to find drugs in cargo containers. R&D might develop ways to use these drug-sniffing dogs to detect explosives or other threatening substances at the same time. If this were possible without reducing the effectiveness of the drug detection, it would be a good example of a dual-use approach that exploits other concerns to further security goals at little added cost or inconvenience. (The use of dogs presents a number of operational challenges, however.)

MITIGATION

Technologies and processes in the "mitigation" category should meet the objective of reducing the harmful impact of an attack as it occurs and in its immediate aftermath. Examples include architectural features that harden a structure against the blast of an explosion, fail-safe or redundant control systems, and protective aerosols that can be sprayed into the air to neutralize chemical agents. Measures of performance specific to this category might include the reduction in damage, casualties, and time out of service.

Biological and Chemical Attacks

There are two main approaches to mitigating the effects of biological and chemical attacks: (1) controlling the dispersal of the agent to prevent or reduce contact with the intended victims and (2) neutralizing or reducing the agent's effectiveness.

Controlling Dispersal

Controlling agent dispersal can mean either designing a system to reduce dispersal-related characteristics in everyday operation or providing active features, such as barriers or ventilation, that would operate only when an attack is detected.

An example of the first approach, platform-edge doors (see Figure 4-1) are fixed panels that fit along the length of a subway platform and remain closed except when a train is in the station loading or unloading passengers. The presence of such a barrier would greatly decrease the piston effect by which trains force contaminated air through tunnels and ventilation systems. Moreover, by slowing the rate at which a biological or chemical agent is dispersed through the system, platform-edge doors would increase the time available for people to escape from the area once an attack was recognized. By reducing the volume of air that must be decontaminated, the existence of a barrier might also reduce the cost and increase the effectiveness of other approaches to mitigation and recovery.

Platform-edge doors are already in use in some locations in Britain, France, Russia, and Singapore, although for reasons having nothing to do with security. (They reduce noise and dust and provide a safety barrier between the tracks and the waiting passengers. These other benefits, in addition to possible security benefits, may help to justify their installation—another example of the dual-use idea.) No platform-edge doors have been installed in U.S. subway systems, but they are similar to the doors used in interterminal transit stations at airports such as Dallas and Atlanta.

This is an existing technology, but there may still be R&D opportunities in investigating its effectiveness at mitigating the impact of biological and chemical

APPLYING THE METHODOLOGY 49

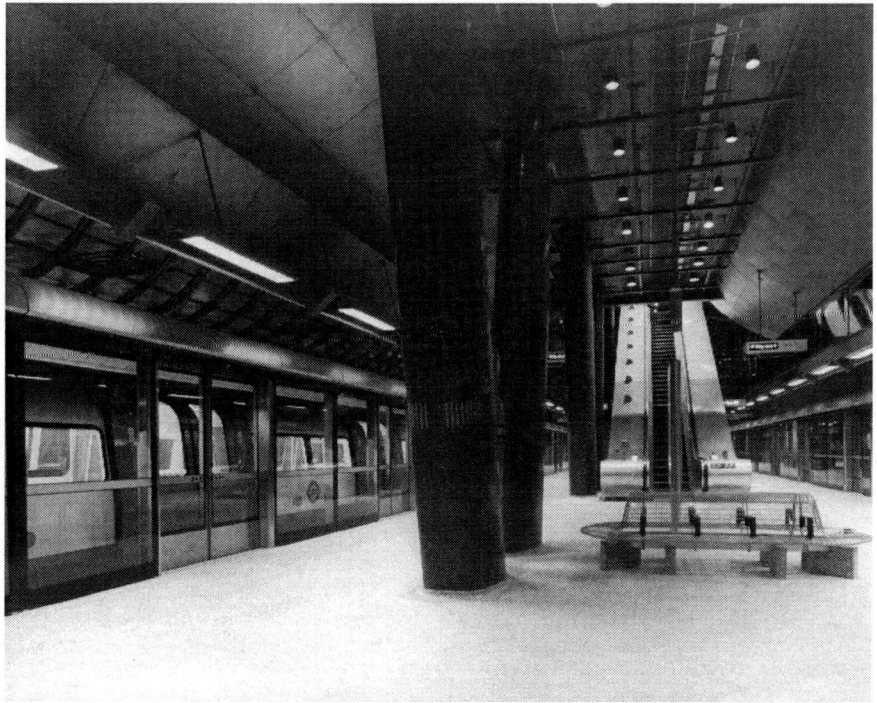

FIGURE 4-1 Platform-edge doors in the London subway. Photo courtesy of Peter Hampshire, London Underground.

attacks, in developing retrofitting techniques for installation in existing subway systems, or simply in adapting and optimizing the technology for use in U.S. subway systems. By its nature, this technology is specific to transportation, so it would be appropriate for DOT's R&D niche.

A variety of active approaches have been proposed for blocking the flow of contaminated air to contain a biological or chemical attack, or alternatively, for ventilating contaminated spaces. These include barrier foams, air curtains, decontamination techniques for the ventilation system, and others, all of which would present R&D opportunities (for details, see Swansiger, 1997). Although these devices could be activated manually, they would be more effective if the existence of detection equipment permitted automated activation. As discussed below under "Monitoring," the synergy with detection technology means that active measures would be more useful for mitigating chemical attacks than biological ones.

Protective Aerosols

In the event of a chemical attack, if immediate escape is impossible, release of a neutralizing agent into the breathing airspace may be the only remedy for people caught in the affected area. Neutralizing aerosols could be developed that would sorb harmful compounds, such as phosphorylating nerve agents, and neutralize them by rapid chemical reactions before they could reach the intended victims. The average specific surface area of an aerosol is hundreds of square meters per gram, which makes aerosol delivery the only flexible way to take rapid remedial action. To provide protection even when the agent used by the attacker is not immediately known, the aerosol chemistry should be designed to counteract a broad spectrum of agents. Sprinkler systems or other mechanisms for dispersing the aerosols would also have to be developed if this option were selected.

Low-Technology Biological and Chemical Protection

A variety of low-technology approaches have been developed to mitigate the consequences of biological or chemical attacks. These include such simple measures as the use of bleach, surgical masks, or simply breathing through a folded t-shirt or wet cloth and moving to a higher location. These are most likely not so much a topic for R&D on the techniques themselves (although some R&D may be necessary to verify their efficacy) as for public education. Thus, here again, DOT's most important role may be identifying, collecting, and disseminating best practices.

Cyber and C^3 Attacks

Among the promising R&D areas for mitigating the consequences of cyber and C^3 attacks specific to surface transportation are ensuring the graceful degradation of damaged or corrupted ITS systems and increasing the robustness of systems that use GPS.

Graceful Degradation of an Intelligent Transportation System

As systems such as ITS become more widespread, centralized controls may create new vulnerabilities to cyber attacks. No doubt the designers of such systems will seek to incorporate fail-safe features, perhaps including hardware features that are redundant with the control software to protect against unanticipated bugs. There are R&D opportunities in ensuring that designs protect against hostile attacks on the central control system as well as against passive failures. One possibility (drawn from the example discussed in Chapter 2) is the development of onboard controls for taking safety measures independently if instructions received from the central system would reduce vehicle headway to an unsafe distance.

The development of redundant or otherwise fault-tolerant system architectures could also contribute to the creation of ITS systems that would degrade gracefully when compromised, either intentionally or otherwise. Such systems would be designed to respond to faults by reducing their functionality in a controlled, planned manner.

In most cases, DOT's role in cyber security is likely to be as a consumer of security technologies and processes, rather than a developer or producer. ITS, however, is a situation unique to transportation that will require particular action.

Interference Mitigation for GPS

The GPS, a satellite-based navigation system originally developed by the Department of Defense, serves marine, airborne, and terrestrial users. There are two GPS services, a civilian one accurate to within 100 meters and a military one accurate to within 20 meters. Enhancements can be used with either service to increase accuracy. One of the primary uses of GPS in surface transportation is determining the location of ships at sea. In addition, GPS receivers are currently being installed in some luxury cars to help identify the fastest route to a destination. As the cost of GPS receivers decreases, the use of GPS in private vehicles is expected to become more widespread.

GPS relies on spread-spectrum signaling, which is inherently robust with respect to low-power interference in the same frequency band. High-power interference from a strategically placed source, however, can easily disrupt the reception of a GPS signal. For example, there has been at least one case of a signal from a military air base inadvertently jamming the reception of a GPS signal by a commercial airplane (Brewin, 1998). This type of threat is likely to become more serious as commercial reliance on GPS signals for positioning and navigation increases. Another concern is the possibility of substituting a false GPS signal that conveys incorrect information. This would require much more sophistication on the part of the attacker, however, than simple jamming.

Sophisticated reception techniques can improve robustness to interference and hostile jamming. For example, if multiple antennas are placed at the receiver, interference that originates from selected locations can be suppressed. The Air Force is currently funding research on a GPS antenna system with this capability (U.S. Air Force, 1998). Additional research on jam-resistant reception techniques for GPS is being supported by the Air Force Office of Scientific Research. DOT should monitor progress in this area and determine whether interference-resistant technologies being developed for air navigation have wider applicability to other modes of (surface) transportation.

Physical Attacks

Analysis of vulnerabilities often leads to the development of new guidelines for structural design. For example, early efforts by the Nuclear Regulatory Commission, working with private industry, postulated various accidents and used the analysis of them to develop design guidelines for licensing nuclear power plants. The commission would postulate broken main steam lines, for example, and the resulting pipe whip would be analyzed to determine the damage to adjacent systems. In this case, the analysis resulted in the development of design methods and requirements for pipe anchors. For surface transportation security, intentional-attack scenarios of varying severity and location would replace accident scenarios. From its work on the vulnerability assessment, DOT already has available many of the tools needed to assess the consequences of an attack, determine the likely damage, and develop protective design enhancements. Box 4-1 highlights some of the design features that might be suggested by

---

Box 4-1
R&D Opportunities in Construction Design

Design Features for Bridges

In California, it is common to see bridge spans that appear to be tied to their supporting abutments by cables. During earthquakes, these tiebacks and other devices help to keep spans from falling off their supports. Tieback systems are likely to be similarly effective against truck bombs under or near a bridge. This simple scheme could be a cheap and effective way to protect critical bridge spans, even in states where seismic resistance is not included in design specifications. Verifying the effectiveness of this approach would require analysis and testing.

Design Features for Tunnels

Engineering reviews are likely to show that most tunnels are quite resistant to explosive damage. Access to urban transit tunnels is usually difficult for an explosive device large enough to cause major damage. Remote tunnels (e.g., railroad tunnels in the wilderness) are more accessible, but even they are probably only susceptible to liner damage, portal damage, and temporary blockage from debris. In many cases, the most significant damage is likely to be to utility lines that run through the tunnel, such as electricity, gas, water, or fuel lines. Tunnels would have to be considered on a case-by-case basis, however, and DOT R&D on analysis techniques could help state and local authorities to perform this task.

Design Features for Pipelines

In some countries, pipeline bombings have become common in recent years. DOT could study these incidents to get a better understanding of the mechanics of such attacks, the resulting damage, and the remedies that have been effective. Communicating the results of this study to domestic pipeline owners and operators through workshops and seminars would not only help them protect their facilities but also heighten their awareness of security concerns.

such an assessment. DOT could also promote the use of such techniques by cities and states, perhaps assisted by the Nunn-Lugar-Domenici program (GAO, 1998).

Analysis of earthquake damage, like analysis of accidents, has led to many new design guidelines. Building code committees, first formed in the 1930s following the first studies of earthquake forces and how structures respond to them, continue to improve seismic design methods and reduce property damage and loss of life. Research continues to contribute by improving our understanding of the regional and magnitude distribution of earthquakes. Fewer cases of damage from intentional attack are available for study, but just as new knowledge has benefited seismic design, the study of past hostile incidents could be used to guide research directions and code development.

It may be decided that design guidelines for protection against explosions should be kept confidential and not incorporated into building codes. For example, the designs of many blast-resistant and defensive military structures are based on Defense Department technical handbooks rather than civilian building codes. The recommendations in these handbooks are the result of years of military research on explosives and penetrators—a reminder of DOT's opportunity to capitalize on the extensive security R&D already conducted by other agencies.

At least one off-the-shelf software package already exists for analyzing the structural effects of an explosion. It incorporates a three-dimensional model of the structure itself along with the spatial position and energy of the explosive device, and it predicts the damage caused to each structural element by the blast. Research by DOT may be needed to modify such tools for analysis of transportation-related structures or to identify and extend other tools already available in other agencies. DOT could also conduct field tests or other research to calibrate models against actual results on transportation structures.

MONITORING

Technologies and processes in the "monitoring" category should meet the objective of recognizing when an attack is under way, characterizing it, and predicting and monitoring its development. Examples include real-time chemical detection systems and intrusion-monitoring software.

Generally Applicable Techniques

Video monitoring, which has already been discussed in the context of identifying imminent attacks, could also be useful in monitoring the course of an attack that has already begun.

Video surveillance requires high-bandwidth communications between the camera and the monitor. These links are often dedicated wires, but they may also be wireless, particularly for cameras on buses and trains. For monitors connected via a local-area network, which may be an attractive approach for buses and trains, R&D could determine data rates and data traffic characteristics, which would dictate the size of digital transmission facilities and the resulting quality of service.

Video surveillance could also be used to complement other monitoring techniques. The problem of false alarms by chemical detectors is a good example. Strategically placed cameras, coupled with event detection and recognition software, might enable a human operator to confirm quickly that a real attack is under way and to initiate evacuation and mitigation procedures. R&D may be needed to identify effective ways to achieve such synergies.

Biological and Chemical Attacks

Detecting Chemical Attacks in Progress

To minimize the effects of a chemical attack, remedial action must be taken quickly, so real-time detection systems are important. Ideally, a system should sound an alarm before the chemical agent reaches its target. If this is not possible, a quick alarm at the same time as the first casualties would at least prevent additional potential victims from entering the area. As noted in Chapter 3, a number of detection systems for chemical agents have already been developed, but their application in transportation environments such as subway systems presents many challenging problems. The acceptable rate of false alarms is very low in a subway, even in comparison with other large civilian facilities, because even if just one train or station is affected directly, that localized disruption is likely to disrupt operations system-wide. Practical detectors must remain functional during long standby periods. They must respond quickly, probably in about one second or less. They must detect a wide variety of agents, ideally based on their physiological impact rather than a predetermined list of chemicals, much as a smoke detector detects "smoke" without knowing its chemical composition.

Given these requirements, an R&D role for DOT may be to evaluate the performance of available detectors in subway use. DOT is not, and should not attempt to be, a leader in the development of new detection technology.

Detecting Biological Attacks in Progress

If practical biological detectors became available, much of the discussion above would also apply to detecting biological attacks. The availability of biological detectors seems highly unlikely, however, in the foreseeable future.

Understanding this judgment requires understanding the differences between detectors and assays. Detectors must operate continuously, whereas assays are conducted during a finite period of time in several discrete, discontinuous steps, such as sample preparation, reagent mixing, incubation, separation, and counting.

Although most modern biological assays are automated, there is always a time delay between the introduction of a sample into the system and the actual acquisition of information. The total required time for a biological assay is typically measured in hours, which is too long to be useful for identifying biological attacks in progress. (Automated assays might be useful in the aftermath of an attack, however, as discussed below.)

How can DOT determine whether biological assays would meet its needs? As usual, answering this question requires evaluating the technology's performance against the objectives of its intended application. For example, if passengers on a train were exposed to a germ warfare agent, symptoms would probably develop hours later, perhaps days later, but to be of value in preventing exposure, positive identification of the agent would have to be made within seconds of the release. DOT's needs would therefore require an information acquisition rate much faster than assays can provide. A second objective would almost certainly be continuous unattended operation, which is hard to imagine for even the most automated assay systems.

The committee is not aware of any detector for biological agents that meets these criteria, or even of any principle on which such a detector could be based. In a number of current R&D efforts (most of them sponsored by the Department of Defense), biological assays are mislabeled as biological sensors or detectors. This mislabeling should not be allowed to create the false impression that direct, continuous, rapid detection of biological agents is possible, let alone imminent.

Baseline Measurements of Chemical and Biological Traces in Subways

The confined air in an urban subway is likely to be a very difficult background against which to identify either toxic chemicals or harmful microorganisms. Baseline measurements of normal levels of chemical and biological traces, as a guide for the development or selection of detection systems, might be a useful R&D project and would clearly be specific to transportation. However, because real-time detection of biological agents is not foreseeable under any background conditions, the focus of baseline measurements should be on the chemical background. (Although unlikely to contribute to real-time detection, measurements of the biological background might be useful after an incident in conjunction with biological assays during the recovery and investigation phase.)

Automated Field Assays, Stand-Off Sensors, and Rapid Off-Site Identification

Although existing biological and chemical analytical assay systems are too slow or not sufficiently automated to operate as detection systems, they can be automated for use in the field. For chemical attacks, there are also stand-off sensing systems for identifying the nature, quantity, and concentration of a chemical agent. Automated field assays and stand-off sensors could help emergency personnel identify the nature of an attack (or apparent attack) in the immediate aftermath of a release.

Micromechanical structures have made the miniaturization and automation of these procedures more economical and even portable. Applications include DNA analysis, gene detection, immunoassays, and toxin assays. The Department of Defense has invested heavily in programs to develop these systems, and this investment has produced some very impressive results. The resulting systems are assays, however, not detectors.

Rapid off-site identification, say within one or two hours, could play a role similar to that of field assays. That capability would be enhanced by the development of contingency plans for critical locations.

One measure of performance against which to evaluate all of these alternatives might be a "confusion matrix"—a table of estimates of the likelihood of various correct and incorrect identifications, given various chemical and biological samples.

Cyber and C^3 Attacks

Monitoring and detecting intrusions into information systems is a major topic of ongoing research. Most current systems use one of two techniques. Either they seek to recognize known hostile software and attacks, or they attempt to recognize deviations from an expected pattern of behavior. The former may leave the system vulnerable to attacks not previously encountered; the latter may leave the system vulnerable to slow deviations from the norm and to erroneous reactions to unexpected external events. Because transportation C^3 systems are ultimately constrained by the physical characteristics of the transportation network, detecting and monitoring cyber and C^3 attacks may be a more limited and thus more tractable problem in the transportation setting than in general. This may be a promising area for research.

Physical Attacks

Because monitoring responses mostly address the period during an attack, and bomb explosions are by their nature sudden, there appears to be little opportunity for R&D in this category.

RECOVERY

Technologies and processes in the "recovery" category are designed to facilitate rapid reconstitution of services after an attack. Examples include chemical and biological decontamination procedures, backup information systems, plans for rerouting traffic around affected locations, techniques for rapid repair of bridges and roadways, protective clothing and equipment for emergency personnel, and bandwidth reservation and priority schemes to ensure rapid delivery of messages (voice, data, or video) in emergency situations. Measures of performance would include the speed of recovery and the confidence that recovery is complete and robust.

Biological and Chemical Attacks

Other agencies have worked extensively on technologies and processes related to decontamination after a chemical or biological attack. Wash-down procedures, including automated and even robotic systems, are one example. In the past, however, the agents of interest have typically been on a relatively short list of agents believed to be most suitable for military use. Work remains to be done to address other potential agents, such as industrial and agricultural chemicals, that are not in the military class but are still harmful. Besides decontamination, verification that an attack site is truly decontaminated is particularly important for civilian situations such as transportation. When is it considered safe, for example, to reenter a vehicle or facility that has been contaminated? Determining and disseminating advice on best practices for the use of existing equipment may be the most important role here for DOT. Other R&D opportunities might include investigating how facilities could be designed to facilitate decontamination or examining ways to minimize the environmental impact of decontamination procedures on surrounding areas.

Physical Attacks

DOT may have a useful role in adapting rapid bridge and roadway repair techniques, originally developed by the Department of Defense, for civilian use. The key here may simply be to educate potential users about these technologies and make them more easily available to the private sector.

INVESTIGATION

The objective of technologies and processes in the "investigation" category is to determine what happened in an attack, how it happened, and who was responsible. An additional objective is often to answer these questions in a way that can serve as evidence for an eventual prosecution of the perpetrators. The probability of discovery is a likely measure of performance.

Identifying lessons learned from past incidents may be the most suitable subject for DOT's R&D in the investigation category. Some other topics include investigating ways to tag substances that are potential chemical agents or their production precursors; developing forensics teams like those that investigate arsons and bombings; and investigating issues involved in the tagging of explosives. All of these seem more appropriate roles for other agencies than for DOT, however.

As surface transportation makes increasing use of networked information systems, failures in those systems (whether caused by an attack or just an accident) will lead to a need for "cyber forensics." Little is known about how to build networked information and control systems so that they can be analyzed in this fashion. (In contrast, investigators have substantial experience with "black boxes" for airplanes and, more recently, automobiles.) Basic research in system structuring and monitoring will be needed to make this a reality. For example, some mission-critical systems might require logging with write-once storage media. The more basic aspects of this problem may be too widely applicable to be an appropriate task for DOT, but their application to transportation could be appropriate, especially because of the dual-use link with accident safety.

SYSTEMS RESPONSES

Technologies and processes in the "systems responses" category are designed to ensure that other elements of the system function properly together. This category also includes understanding the problem more thoroughly to improve the evaluation and selection of responses in other categories. Because the surface transportation system is so diverse and the problem of protecting it against attack is so complex, there are many opportunities for R&D on systems integration—that is, on integrating technologies and processes across functions and transportation modes to optimize a combination of security and other transportation goals.

Generally Applicable Techniques

A process for "incident management" is already widely used in surface transportation in response to relatively minor incidents—for example, to coordinate the rapid clearing of highway lanes after traffic accidents. This process is mostly a matter of coordination and integration among local governments, police departments, towing companies, and so on. There may be development needs, however, in expanding the concept to broader application in response to intentional attacks. Some similar ideas have already been put in place, under the auspices of the Federal Emergency Management Administration and others, for response to accidental spills of hazardous materials.

A system for reporting incidents and possible incidents would also be valuable. Low-level events—probes rather than actual attacks—may not be reported at all, and if they are, they are likely to be reported in the context of safety rather than security. Thus current reporting mechanisms are not as useful for intelligence purposes as they could be. For example, if there were a repeated pattern of bolt-loosening incidents on railroads, would the railroads share this information with each other and with the intelligence community? Or if there were a pattern of unusual activity in the transportation sector's C^3 systems, would that fact even be identified? Developing a reporting system of this kind would require significant work to identify means of collecting, protecting, and correlating data and to establish criteria for reporting information to the appropriate parties.

Other possibilities include modeling and simulation of organizational responses and coordination, and the development of methods for system-level exercises, training, and public education and communication.

Chemical Attacks

A serious system-level concern for responding to chemical attacks is the lack of understanding of how chemical agents would disperse through a facility under attack. R&D could be conducted to model and experimentally verify the behavior of turbulent chemical plumes, in both closed and open spaces, especially the airflow patterns in specific surface transportation situations, taking into account various passenger loads, weather conditions, and so on. Releases of simulant chemicals could also be studied to help develop response strategies. Dispersion and ventilation could also be addressed more generally. Note that DOT's situation is different from that of the Defense Department because DOT deals primarily with closed spaces (such as vehicles, stations, or tunnels) whereas the Defense Department still deals primarily with open spaces (battlefields). As a result, there are differences between the issues that DOT and the Defense Department need to model and understand, including differences in the agents of concern, their physical properties, and the characteristics of the airflow.

Cyber and C^3 Attacks

DOT could develop best-practices guidelines on computer security for surface transportation providers to help owners and operators learn from each other's experiences. This work would be transportation-specific because best practices for a railroad, for example, are not necessarily the same as best practices for another type of company, such as a bank. The guidelines would not have to become regulations, but they could help to bring transportation companies up to speed on the issues of concern and the state of the art in responding to those issues. The emphasis should be on integrating best practices into everyday operations, making security best practices a component of business best practices. Implementation would require that DOT play a proactive coordinating role in communicating results to the broad transportation community.

The growing and evolving automation of control systems may make surface transportation more and more vulnerable to cyber attacks. For example, supervisory control and data acquisition (SCADA) systems are increasingly being used for the automation or remote control of pipeline operations. Existing commercial technology and research by other agencies could be useful for protecting surface transportation against cyber threats to these systems. An R&D effort in this area by DOT could develop broad guidelines to assist developers of surface transportation infrastructure control systems in making their systems more resistant to cyber attacks. The emphasis should be on ensuring that control systems degrade gracefully, which may require planned redundancy, backup plans, and other measures.

As noted in Chapter 2, a clearer picture of the interdependencies of transportation C^3 systems with other parts of the surface transportation system would be extremely useful.

Finally, control systems could benefit from disaster planning exercises, such as preplanning and modeling. Because control in transportation systems tends to be real-time, test beds distinct from operational systems often already exist, and these could be used to work on disaster planning.

SUMMARY

The R&D topics described in this chapter are intended to illustrate the application of the strategy discussed in Chapter 3. When DOT conducts a more complete and thorough evaluation using that strategy, it may or may not find them to be the highest-priority topics. Nevertheless, four themes are sure to remain:

- the value of taking a *dual-use* approach, in which security objectives are furthered at the same time as other transportation goals
- the potential for more use of *modeling* to improve understanding of the scope of the security problem
- the importance of DOT's role in developing and disseminating information about *best practices* that use existing technologies and processes, including low-technology alternatives
- the need to consider security as *part of a broader picture*, not a wholly new and different problem, but one that is similar and closely connected to the transportation community's previous experience in responding to concerns about safety, natural disasters, and hazardous materials

5

A Vision of the Future

This study's contribution to improving surface transportation security is the first step of a journey. The surface transportation system is remarkably reliable in the face of accidents and natural disasters, but hostile attacks are a different and new concern. Moreover, the pace of technological change is so rapid that, at the same time efforts are made to improve security, dramatic changes are sure to occur in the nature of hostile threats, the vulnerability of transportation to those threats, and the nature of the transportation system itself. The emerging awareness of chemical, biological, and cyber vulnerabilities is just one aspect of the evolution of the security challenge.

In this fluid situation, it will be critical that DOT and other agencies work together in a coherent, unified, but flexible and dynamic way. An effective response will also require the close involvement of many other stakeholders, including the research community, state and local transportation agencies, and above all the owners and operators who provide transportation services across the country. Ensuring this involvement will undoubtedly require overcoming organizational, institutional, and disciplinary barriers.

But although the security of surface transportation is a relatively new concern in one sense, in another sense it is not new at all. Prevention and mitigation of accidents, recovery from natural disasters, and safe handling of hazardous materials are all familiar aspects of the transportation system. Building on this foundation will make enhancing security a more tractable and less daunting task. System designers will have to build security into their plans from the beginning, not add it on at the end. Developers of security features will have to recognize the transportation system's other goals and capitalize on them by selecting dual-use alternatives that benefit transportation owners and operators beyond improved security. Viewing security as part of a broader picture will make the task far easier.

This study has endeavored to identify elements of an R&D strategy for DOT that would further this vision of the future. Some of the report's key findings and recommendations are restated below.

At this early stage in the establishment of an R&D program for surface transportation security, building a solid strategic basis is the most important task. The strategy should be a systematic process consisting of five fundamental steps:

1. *Defining* the problem, the objectives, and the criteria for evaluating success or failure
2. *Identifying* ways to meet the objectives, namely potential R&D projects
3. *Evaluating* the alternatives identified in Step 2 against the objectives defined in Step 1
4. *Deciding* on a course of action
5. *Implementing* the decision

The implementation of this strategy should incorporate the following key features:

- Because improving security is a crosscutting problem, DOT should not break up its efforts in this area according to transportation modes.
- DOT should clearly identify and understand its role in security R&D and how that role meshes with work being done by other agencies.
- As a framework for identifying and evaluating potential R&D topics, DOT should categorize topics according to the type of attack to which they respond and the type of response to which they are directed: prevention, mitigation, monitoring, recovery, investigation, or systems.
- DOT should make strenuous efforts to increase the involvement of transportation owners and operators. Their serious involvement in all stages of the program will be critical to successful implementation.
- To meet the growing need to protect information that is sensitive, but not classified, DOT should consider urging the Congress to provide legal authority similar to the regulation 14 CFR 191, which protects information on aviation security.

Vulnerability assessment is an important part of defining the security problem in Step 1 above. DOT has already made commendable progress in this area. Those efforts should be continued, with attention to the following points:

- further checking of the basic assumptions and predicted consequences of attack scenarios, in cooperation with experts from industry

- further assessment of threat likelihood, where possible
- a more complete, balanced, and clearly defined analysis of possible means of attack
- more attention to cyber attacks and other attacks on C^3 systems, especially attacks other than the introduction of computer viruses
- a close examination of chemical and biological vulnerabilities
- careful distinction between chemical attacks and biological attacks and between attacks involving agents with different properties
- an examination of strategic, systemic vulnerabilities

To improve its understanding of strategic vulnerabilities, DOT should undertake (1) a strategic assessment of the surface transportation system's redundancies and interdependencies, and (2) an analysis of lessons learned about impact and mitigation from past accidents and natural disasters.

When DOT conducts a complete and thorough evaluation of potential R&D topics, using this systematic five-step strategy, the following themes will emerge:

- the value of taking a *dual-use* approach, in which security objectives are furthered at the same time as other transportation goals
- the potential for more use of *modeling* to improve understanding of the scope of the security problem
- the importance of DOT's role in developing and disseminating information about *best practices* that use existing technologies and processes, including low-technology alternatives
- the need to consider security as *part of a broader picture*, not a wholly new and different problem, but one that is similar and closely connected to the transportation community's previous experience in responding to concerns about safety, natural disasters, and hazardous materials

References

Aymeric, M. 1999. Personal communication from M. Aymeric, Department of Transport (France), to D. Morgan, June 8, 1999.

Brewin, B. 1998. Rogue transmitter knocks out GPS signals. Federal Computer Week 12(10): 1.

CIAO (Critical Infrastructure Assurance Office). 1998. Preliminary Research and Development Roadmap for Protecting and Assuring Critical National Infrastructures. Washington, D.C.: Critical Infrastructure Assurance Office.

Davis, J. 1998. Presentation to the Committee on R&D Strategies to Improve Surface Transportation Security, Washington, D.C., November 4, 1998.

DOT (U.S. Department of Transportation). 1998a. Surface Transportation Vulnerability Assessment (classified document). Washington, D.C.: U.S. Department of Transportation.

DOT. 1998b. Worldwide Terrorism and Violent Criminal Attacks Against Transportation—1996. Background paper prepared for this study. Washington, D.C.: Office of Intelligence and Security, U.S. Department of Transportation.

DOT. 1999a. DOT Budget in Brief—FY 2000. Washington, D.C.: U.S. Department of Transportation.

DOT. 1999b. FY 2000 President's Budget, Budget Authority Table for Research, Development and Technology, January 28, 1999. Washington, D.C.: U.S. Department of Transportation.

GAO (General Accounting Office). 1997. Combating Terrorism: Spending on Governmentwide Programs Requires Better Management and Coordination. GAO/NSIAD-98-39. Washington, D.C.: General Accounting Office.

GAO. 1998. Combating Terrorism. GAO/NSIAD-98-74. Washington, D.C.: General Accounting Office.

Giuliano, G., and J. Golob. 1998. Impacts of the Northridge earthquake on transit and highway use. Journal of Transportation and Statistics 1(2): 1–20.

Gordon, P., H.W. Richardson, and B. Davis. 1998. Transport related impacts of the Northridge earthquake. Journal of Transportation and Statistics 1(2): 21–36.

Henderson, D.A. 1999. The looming threat of bioterrorism. Science 283: 1279–1282.

REFERENCES

IOM and NRC (Institute of Medicine and National Research Council). 1999. Chemical and Biological Terrorism: Research and Development to Improve Civilian Medical Response. Washington, D.C.: National Academy Press.

Keeney, R.L., and H. Raiffa. 1976. Decisions with Multiple Objectives: Preferences and Value Trade-Offs. New York: John Wiley and Sons.

Mineta Institute (Norman Y. Mineta International Institute for Surface Transportation Policy Studies). 1997. Protecting Surface Transportation Systems and Patrons from Terrorist Activities: Case Studies of Best Security Practices and a Chronology of Attacks. San Jose, Calif.: San Jose State University.

Neifert, A. 1996. Case study: sarin poisoning of subway passengers in Tokyo, Japan, in March, 1995. Medical NBC Information Server of the U.S. Army Medical Department (posted August 2, 1996). http://www.nbcmed.org/csjapan.html.

NRC (National Research Council). 1998. Trust in Cyberspace. Washington, D.C.: National Academy Press.

NRC. 1999. Final Report of the Committee on Commercial Aviation Security. National Materials Advisory Board. In progress.

Ohbu, S., A.Yamashina, N. Takasu, T. Yamaguchi, T. Murai, K. Nakano, Y. Matsui, R. Mikami, K. Sakurai, and S. Hinohara. 1997. Sarin poisoning on Tokyo subway. Southern Medical Journal 90(6): 587–593.

PCCIP (Presidential Commission on Critical Infrastructure Protection). 1997. Critical Foundations: Protecting America's Infrastructures. Washington, D.C.: Government Printing Office. Available on the Internet at www.pccip.gov/report_index.html.

Swansiger, W.A. 1997. Defending Subways Against Chem-Bio Terrorism. SAND 98-8210. Livermore, Calif.: Sandia National Laboratories.

Thompson, K. 1984. Reflections on trusting trust (half of the 1983 Turing Award lecture). Communications of the ACM 27: 761–764.

U.S. Air Force. 1998. Internet home page of the GAS-1 GPS antenna system. http://gps.laafb.af.mil/user/products/gas-1/ (update of October 30, 1998).

U.S. Department of State. 1997. Patterns of Global Terrorism 1996. 10433. Washington, D.C.: U.S. Department of State.

Weinstein, B.L., and T.L. Clower. 1998. The impacts of the Union Pacific service disruptions on the Texas and national economies: an unfinished story. Report to the Railroad Commission of Texas, February 9, 1998. http://www.rrc.state.tx.us/divisions/rail/UPFINAL3.html.

Appendices

Appendix A

Background on Systems Theory

Over the past 50 years or so, researchers have built up a considerable literature on systems theory that includes both theoretical perspectives and case studies of specific applications. DOT should capitalize on this work in establishing its process for selecting and funding R&D projects in surface transportation security. Because the systems engineering literature may be unfamiliar to many readers, this appendix briefly summarizes some key points and provides a few references for further reading. This discussion is not meant to provide a complete survey of the literature.

Kahneman, Slovic, and Tversky (1982) showed clearly that unaided decision making is fraught with numerous biases. A systematic methodology provides some protection against these biases. Much of the early work on systems engineering focused on techniques rather than methodology (see, for example, Morse and Kimball, 1950). In some ways, the successes of systems engineering and operations research during and immediately after World War II, primarily in military projects, impeded the development of a formal methodology (see Hall, 1989). However, by the late 1950s and 1960s a number of systems thinkers had begun to define overriding methodologies rather than focusing on specific techniques (e.g., Churchman et al., 1957; Hall, 1962; Ackoff et al., 1962; and Churchman, 1968).

At the heart of these methodologies were five steps: problem definition, generation of alternatives, evaluation, decision, and implementation. These are the same five stages described in Chapter 3 in the recommended R&D strategy for surface transportation security. The steps are typically taken in sequence, but results may sometimes require going back to a previous step. Backwards motion does not necessarily mean failure. For example, problems that consist of several phases may require several passes through the sequence, so that each phase can incorporate feedback from earlier phases.

The five-step methodology matches closely with the rational decision-making model studied by economists and political scientists, an approach that was discredited as a descriptive model for organizations and economics by March and Simon (1958) and for political decision making by Allison (1971). In systems engineering, however, the methodology is intended to be normative rather than descriptive. Moreover, the systems engineering context lacks the computational and organizational limitations that social scientists highlighted for practical economic and political situations.

Recent work has focused on extending the basic approach. Many situations, especially large defense projects, require consideration of legal and contractual issues in addition to technological evaluation (Blanchard, 1998, and DOD, 1996). The nature of complexity and the search for general approaches to describing it have altered some features of the basic approach (Albin and Foley, 1998). Several researchers have developed and employed "soft" methodologies for working with problems that have loose, ill-structured, or ill-defined specifications (Checkland and Scholes, 1990). The methodology described in the body of this report relies primarily on the basic methodology without these recent additions, but extensions could be accommodated easily.

REFERENCES

Ackoff, R.L., S.K. Gupta, and J.S. Minas. 1962. Scientific Method: Optimizing Applied Research Questions. New York: John Wiley and Sons.
Albin, P.S., and D.K. Foley, eds. 1998. Barriers and Bounds to Rationality: Essays on Economic Complexity and Dynamics in Interactive Systems. Princeton, N.J.: Princeton University Press.
Allison, G.T. 1971. The Essence of Decision. Boston: Little Brown.
Blanchard, B. 1998. Systems Engineering Management. 2nd ed. New York: John Wiley and Sons.
Checkland, P., and J. Scholes. 1990. Soft Systems Methodology in Action. New York: John Wiley and Sons.
Churchman, C.W. 1968. The Systems Approach. New York: Delacorte.
Churchman, C.W., R.L. Ackoff, and E.L. Arnoff. 1957. Introduction to Operations Research. New York: John Wiley and Sons.
DOD (U.S. Department of Defense). 1996. Mandatory Procedures for Major Defense Acquisition Programs (MDAPs) and Major Automated Information System (MAIS) Acquisition Programs. DODR 5000.2-R. Washington, D.C.: U.S. Department of Defense.
Hall, A.D. 1962. A Methodology for Systems Engineering. New York: Van Nostrand.
Hall, A.D. 1989. Metasystems Methodology: A New Synthesis and Unification. Oxford, U.K.: Pergamon.
Kahneman, D., P. Slovic, and A. Tversky. 1982. Judgment Under Uncertainty: Heuristics and Biases. Cambridge, U.K.: Cambridge University Press.
March, J., and P. Simon. 1958. Organizations. New York: John Wiley and Sons.
Morse, P.M., and G.E. Kimball. 1950. Methods of Operations Research. New York: John Wiley and Sons.

APPENDIX B

The Likely Course of Development of Chemical and Biological Attacks

Figures B-1 and B-2 may help to clarify the important differences between chemical and biological attacks. They are reproduced from (IOM and NRC, 1999).

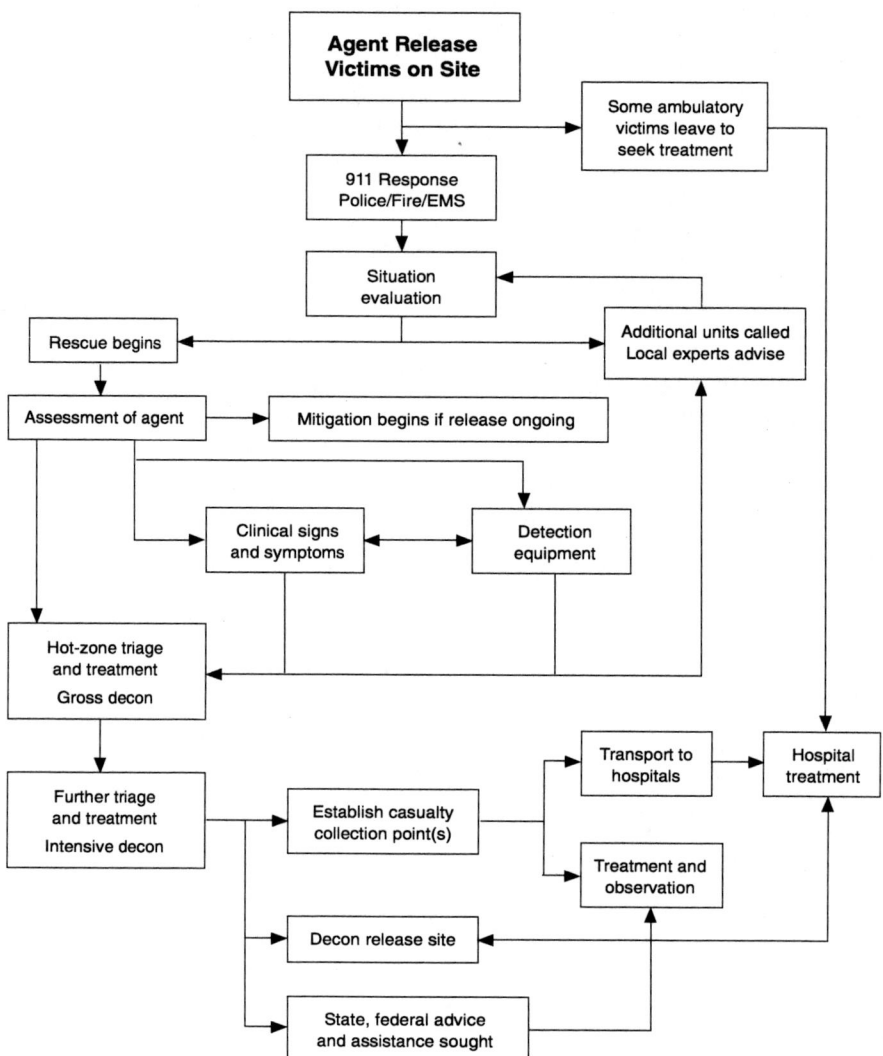

FIGURE B-1 Flow chart of probable actions in a chemical agent incident.

APPENDIX B

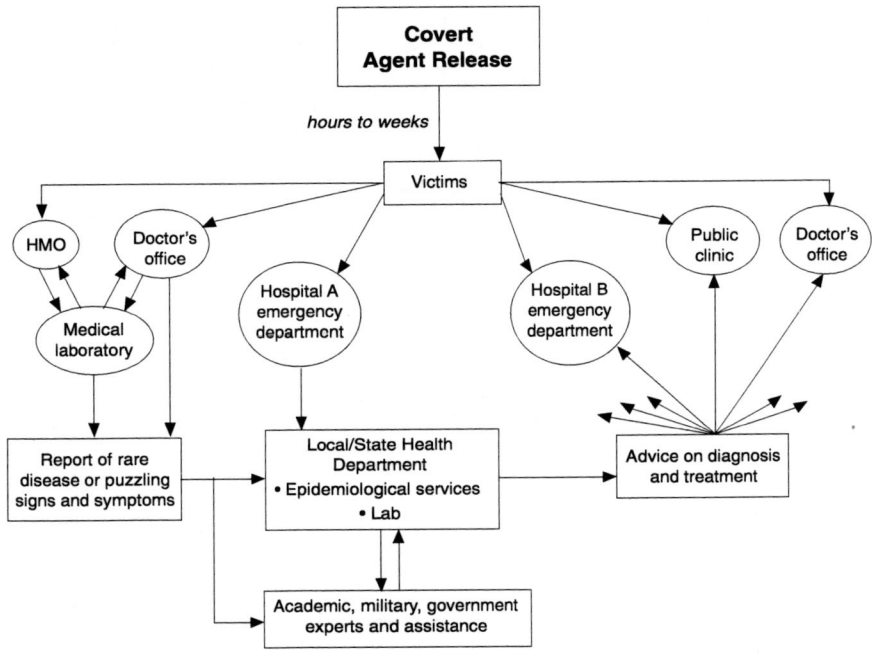

FIGURE B-2 Flow chart of probable actions in a biological agent incident.

REFERENCE

IOM and NRC (Institute of Medicine and National Research Council). 1999. Chemical and Biological Terrorism: Research and Development to Improve Civilian Medical Response. Washington, D.C.: National Academy Press.

Biographical Sketches of Committee Members

H. Norman Abramson *(chair)* is executive vice president (retired) of Southwest Research Institute. He is internationally known in the field of applied mechanics, particularly for his expertise in the dynamics of contained liquids, and he has extensive experience working on issues involving technology transfer and transportation. He has served as an officer or director of several professional societies, including the American Society of Mechanical Engineers and the American Institute of Aeronautics and Astronautics. He is a member of the National Academy of Engineering (NAE) and served on the NAE Council from 1984 to 1990. He has served on more than 20 committees of the NAE and the National Research Council (NRC), including the Committee on the Federal Transportation R&D Strategic Planning Process, which he chaired.

Donald E. Brown is chair of the Department of Systems Engineering of the University of Virginia. His research focuses on data fusion and simulation optimization with applications to intelligence, security, logistics, and transportation. He has developed decision support systems for several U.S. intelligence agencies and was previously an intelligence operations officer for the U.S. Army. Dr. Brown is coeditor of *Operations Research and Artificial Intelligence: The Integration of Problem Solving Strategies* (Kluwer Academic Publishers, 1990) and *Intelligent Scheduling Systems* (Kluwer Academic Publishers, 1995) and is an associate editor for the journal *International Abstracts in Operations Research*. He has been president, vice president, and secretary of the Systems, Man, and Cybernetics Society of the Institute of Electrical and Electronics Engineers (IEEE). He is past chairman of the Technical Section on Artificial Intelligence of the Institute for Operations Research and Management Science and was awarded that society's Outstanding Service Award.

Nick Cartwright is officer in charge of the Science and Technology Branch of the Royal Canadian Mounted Police (RCMP) and manager of the Canadian Police Research Centre, a partnership of the RCMP, the Canadian Association of Chiefs of Police, and the National Research Council of Canada. He is an expert in the development and use of technology in law enforcement and crime solution. He serves on the advisory council of the U.S. Justice Department that reviews and analyzes the technological needs of the criminal justice system. He chairs the International Civil Aviation Organization's Ad Hoc Group of Specialists on the Detection of Explosives and is a member of the scientific advisory panel that reviews and oversees the security R&D program of the U.S. Federal Aviation Administration. He is a member of the steering committee of Transport Canada's Security Screening Equipment Project and cochair of its working group on standards and technology.

A. Ray Chamberlain, a civil engineer, is a transportation consultant and area manager for Parsons Brinckerhoff. Until recently, he was the vice president for freight policy of the American Trucking Associations (ATA). In that position he served as the ATA's liaison to the Presidential Commission on Critical Infrastructure Protection (PCCIP). He has held several other senior positions in private industry, state government, and academia and has been president of both the American Association of State Highway and Transportation Officials and the National Association of State Universities and Land Grant Colleges. He chaired the executive committee of the NRC Transportation Research Board in 1993 and has served on numerous NRC committees, including the Committee on the Federal Transportation R&D Strategic Planning Process.

H. Andy Franklin, principal engineer with the R&D department of Bechtel Technology, Inc., has project engineering and management experience in the design, analysis, testing, and construction of a wide range of industrial facilities, systems, and machinery. His expertise includes structural forensics for damaged and failed facilities, as well as inspection and recovery of facilities after major earthquakes. Dr. Franklin's recent work includes the development of a unique steel-fiber concrete with very high tensile strength for use in applications subject to shock loading (such as bomb blasts). He is a member of the American Concrete Institute and the American Society of Civil Engineers (ASCE) and was recently chair of the ASCE Aerospace Division.

Robert E. Green, Jr., is director of the Center for Nondestructive Evaluation, professor in the Materials Science and Engineering Department, and member of the principal professional staff at the Applied Physics Laboratory of The Johns

Hopkins University. His experience includes previous positions in both industry and government. He has served on several NRC committees, the board of directors of the American Society for Nondestructive Testing (ASNT) of which he is currently president, the advisory board of *Materials Technology*, and the editorial board of *Research in Nondestructive Evaluation*. He is an active member of numerous professional societies, a fellow of both ASM International and ASNT, and cofounder of the International Symposium on Nondestructive Characterization of Materials.

Bruce Haddan is assistant vice president for applied technology at Norfolk Southern Corporation, where his responsibilities include security, disaster recovery, data warehousing, industrial engineering, operations research, and advanced technology. He has also held positions at Norfolk Southern in the auditing, accounting, and information technology departments and in a trucking subsidiary, North American Van Lines. He chaired a subcommittee of the American National Standards Institute committee on electronic data interchange during its development and issuance of standards for encryption and authentication. He has also served on and chaired numerous committees and subcommittees of the Association of American Railroads.

William J. Harris is a metallurgist with extensive experience in the railroad industry. He served on the PCCIP and is currently a consultant to the Critical Infrastructure Assurance Office. He is an emeritus professor of transportation engineering at Texas A&M University and has held a variety of other research and transportation-related positions in government and the private sector. He has served as president of the Metallurgical Society, president of the Engineers Joint Council, honorary board member of ITS America, member of the executive committee of the NRC Transportation Research Board, and organizer and president of the International Heavy Haul Association. He is a member of the NAE.

Michael L. Honig, the Ameritech Professor of Information Technology at Northwestern University, has expertise in data transmission and reception and wireless communication networks. He previously spent 13 years at Bell Laboratories and Bellcore working on voice-band data transmission, local-area networks, digital subscriber lines, and wireless communications. He is coauthor of the book *Adaptive Filters: Structures, Algorithms, and Applications* (Kluwer Academic Publishers, 1984) and has served as editor and guest editor for a number of international journals. He is a fellow of the IEEE and a member of the board of governors of its Information Theory Society.

Jiri (Art) Janata is professor of chemistry at the Georgia Institute of Technology. His research includes analytical chemistry, electrochemistry, chemical sensors, bioinstrumentation, biophysical chemistry, fundamentals of materials science, micromachining, and instrumental analysis. He was previously associate director for materials and interfaces in the Environmental Molecular Science Laboratory at Pacific Northwest National Laboratory. He has organized and chaired numerous symposia and conferences. He is on the editorial boards of *Biosensors*, *Sensor Technology*, and *Talanta* and the advisory board of *Analytical Chemistry* and is an associate editor for *Field Analytical Chemistry and Technology*.

Steven B. Lipner is director of the Systems Technology Center division of Mitretek Systems, which specializes in software engineering, Internet and client-server technology, computer and network security, and software and project economics and costing. He is also chair of Mitretek's corporate information security committee and sponsored research committee. Previously he was a vice president at Trusted Information Systems, director of information systems in the Center for Information Systems of MITRE Corporation, and manager of the Secure Systems Group at Digital Equipment Corporation. He was a member of the National Computer Systems Security and Privacy Advisory Board from 1989 to 1993.

Michael D. Meyer is chair of the School of Civil and Environmental Engineering at the Georgia Institute of Technology. Previously he was the director of transportation planning and development for the state of Massachusetts and before that a professor of civil engineering at the Massachusetts Institute of Technology. He has published more than 120 technical articles and authored or coauthored numerous texts on transportation planning and policy. He is active in professional organizations, consulting, and expert review panels at the national, state, and local levels. His particular interests in transportation policy include the implementation process, the cost effectiveness of investments, and performance measures.

Fred V. Morrone is director of public safety and superintendent of police for the Port Authority of New York and New Jersey, which operates some of the nation's largest and busiest transportation facilities, including airports, port terminals, toll bridges, tunnels, bus and rail transit systems, and the World Trade Center. As head of the 1,300-member Department of Public Safety, he is responsible for planning, developing, implementing, and administering the Port Authority's police and fire services. He has more than 35 years of experience in security and is a member of the American Society for Industrial Security and the New Jersey, New York, and International Associations of Chiefs of Police. He is a member of the latter's Subcommittee on Terrorism.

Julia Weertman is a professor of materials science and engineering at Northwestern University. Her research is focused on the mechanical behavior of metals and alloys, deformation mechanisms, and microstructural characterization. She has served on numerous university advisory boards and federal advisory committees and is a fellow of both the Minerals, Metals, and Materials Society and ASM International. She is a member of the NAE and has served on a wide variety of NAE and NRC committees, including the NAE Council and the NRC Solid State Sciences Committee, of which she is a former chair.